The Medical Dictionary for Bad Spellers

The Medical Dictionary for Bad Spellers

Joseph Krevisky and **Jordan L. Linfield**

An Innovation Press Book

John Wiley & Sons, Inc.

New York • Chichester • Brisbane • Toronto • Singapore

This text is printed on acid-free paper.

Copyright © 1995 by Innovation Press
Published by John Wiley & Sons, Inc.

All rights reserved. Published simultaneously in Canada.

This publication is designed to provide accurate and authoritative information in regard to the subject matter covered. It is sold with the understanding that the publisher is not engaged in rendering professional services. If legal, accounting, medical, psychological, or any other expert assistance is required, the services of a competent professional person should be sought.

ISBN 0-471-31069-7

Printed in the United States of America

10 9 8 7 6 5 4 3 2 1

Contents

Introduction

"If I don't know how to spell the word, how can I find it in the dictionary?"
This lament has been the subject of cartoons, comic strips, columns by popular writers, TV sitcoms, and radio talk shows.

"It doesn't look right." Sound familiar? Most of us, regardless of age or education, face this problem sometimes, or often. Poor spelling has little to do with intelligence, level of schooling, family background, or heredity. Presidents and princes, Ph.D.'s and M.D.'s, poets and professors all boast bad spellers within their groups. In fact, boast is often what these poor spellers do; they are proud of it.

Why, then, is bad spelling such a widespread problem?

The major cause is the complex pattern of English spelling and pronunciation. For example, the same letter may be pronounced several different ways. Note the pronunciation of the letter *c*

in the word *cell* (pronounced as an *s*)
in the word *callus* (pronounced as a *k*)
in the word *alopecia* (pronounced as *sh*)
in the word *cello* (pronounced as *ch*)

And sometimes it is silent, as in the words *yacht, Connecticut,* and *czar.* To add to the confusion, some words are spelled alike but pronounced differently: Note the word *wound*, meaning injury, is pronounced "woond," and the word *wound*, as in a clock, is pronounced "waund."

Some words are pronounced alike but are spelled and defined differently:

calculus and *calculous*
caul and *call*
ameleia and *amelia*
filum and *phylum*

Some words are pronounced and spelled almost alike but are defined differently:

enervate and *innervate*

aerogenous and *erogenous*

Our medical language is further complicated by the extensive use of Greek and Latin terms, particularly prefixes and suffixes.

Spelling errors in medicine can have serious consequences—much more serious than the embarrassment or inconvenience of finding a wrong spelling in everyday life. So what? After all, a computer spell-checker does the work. It will quickly spot a misspelled word and provide the correct spelling.

Or will it?

First, you must be sure—even with simple misspellings—that you choose the right word from the options offered by the PC.

Second, many spell-checkers do not include words that have come into our language recently, such as *fax* or *nymble*.

Third, and this is surprising, the typical computer used in hospitals and medical offices contains very few medical terms. It is unlikely that your spell-checker contains the word *cyst*, let alone *sebaceous*. Above all, no computer can catch the differences between words that look alike or sound alike. The computer cannot indicate the correct usage of *their*, *there*, or *they're*. The computer will provide the options but the choice is thrown back to you. So you are unlikely to get any help if you misuse *discuss* for *discous* or *distall* for *distill*.

And what do you do when you don't have a PC handy, for instance, when you are traveling, in the library, or when the computer is down?

The Medical Dictionary for Bad Spellers solves these problems. It provides an extensive list of words that are typically misspelled—both medical and general terminology—in alphabetical order by their misspellings. Look the word up by its misspelling and you will find the correct spelling alongside it. The misspelled words are listed by their obvious misspelling: for example, *cenile* for *senile*. More difficult words are listed by several variant misspellings to increase your chances of finding them speedily.

The corpus of this dictionary, with its wide variety of misspellings, has been collected by the authors during years of working on the vagaries of English and in compiling popular dictionaries. *The Medical Dictionary for Bad Spellers* also provides the only available list of medical look-alikes and sound-alikes, which are sources of increasing confusion in our medical writings. And finally, there is a handy quick list of correct spellings for reference if you are reasonably sure of the spelling.

Of particular value is the inclusion of an extensive list of prefixes and suffixes in Section 1, Words Arranged by Their Common Misspellings. Medical terminology is built, to a large degree, on Greek and Latin affixes. Thus, a typical prefix such as *cyto-* combines with nearly 100 words. *Cyto-*

is listed in Section 1 alongside the incorrect spellings *sito-* and *syto-*. It is also listed in Section 3, Quick List of Correct Spellings. So, whether you know how to spell *cyto-* correctly or incorrectly, you can find it easily. And you have immediate entrée to nearly 100 additional words.

Prefixes are indicated by a hyphen at the end (e.g., *cyto-*). Suffixes are indicated by a hyphen at the beginning (e.g., *-phobia*). In both cases, when the combining affix is used in a word, the hyphen is dropped, as in *cytoscope* or *hydrophobia*.

How to Use This Dictionary

The Medical Dictionary for Bad Spellers is arranged in three parts. Section 1, Words Arranged by their Common Misspellings, consists of words arranged alphabetically by their incorrect spellings, with the correct spelling in the opposite column. Section 2, Words Commonly Confused Because they Look Alike or Sound Alike, comprises a list of words that look alike or sound alike, with brief definitions illustrating the differences. Section 3 is the Quick List of Correct Spellings.

If you are reasonably sure of the spelling of a word, check it in the alphabetical Quick List of Correct Spellings. If you do not find it there, check Section 1—the list of incorrect spellings with their correct spellings. Try the phonetic spelling *sistoscopy* for *cystoscopy*, for example. Once you have found the correct spelling, be sure to look over the entire correct word carefully; while we emphasize misspellings at the beginnings of words, we include standard middle and ending errors such as *site* for *cyte,* as in *melanosite* for *melanocyte*; or *sine* for *cine*, as in *glysine* for *glycine*. When asterisks (**) appear next to the correct spelling of a word in either Section 1 or Section 3, the word should be checked as a look-alike or sound-alike in Section 2, as this is a word that looks like or sounds like another word and is apt to be misused.

Suppose, for example, you are not sure how to spell *geranial*. You think it is spelled *gerranial*. You look it up in Section 3, the Quick List of Correct Spellings. You do not find it there. Turning to Section 1, Words Arranged by Their Common Misspellings, you look up *gerranial* in the list of incorrect spellings and find it along with the correct spelling, *geranial***. The asterisks alert you to check Section 2, Words Commonly Confused Because They Look Alike or Sound Alike. This section shows you the difference between *geranial* and *geraniol*. The latter word may be the one you sought in the first place.

SECTION 1

Words Arranged by Their Common Misspellings

A

abaration .... aberration
abarent .... aberrant
abb- (pre) .... ab-
abbdomen .... abdomen
abbducens nerve ...... abducens nerve
abbduct .... abduct
abbducter .... abductor**
abbiojenesis .... abiogenesis
abblatio .... ablatio**
abblation .... ablation**
abbnormal behavior ....
.... abnormal behavior
abbortifacient .... abortifacient
abbortin .... abortin**
abbrasion .... abrasion
abbrasive .... abrasive
abbruptio .... abruptio
abbsission .... abscission
abbsorb .... absorb**
abbsorption .... absorption
abbulia .... abulia
abcess .... abscess
ABC pouder .... ABC powder
abdomminal cavity ....
.... abdominal cavity
abdukter .... abductor**
-abel (suff) .... -able
abelled .... abled
abeojenesis .... abiogenesis
aberation .... aberration
abliteration .... obliteration
abnormallity .... abnormality
abnorrmal psychology ....
.... abnormal psychology
aborshion .... abortion**
abo system .... ABO system
absalute .... absolute
absess .... abscess
absorrptive state ...... absorptive state
abstanense .... abstinence
abstetrical .... obstetrical
abstipation .... obstipation
abyuse .... abuse
acclusal .... occlusal
accoostic nerve ...... acoustic nerve

acctinobacillus .... actinobacillus
acctive hyperemia ....
.... active hyperemia
-ace (suff) .... -ase
aceetal .... acetal**
acettiminifen .... acetaminophen
ackapnia .... acapnia**
ackeous .... aqueous
acklusive .... occlusive
acknee .... acne
ackrid .... acarid**
ackson .... axon**
acommodation .... accommodation
acshion potential ...... action potential
acson transport ...... axon transport
acth .... ACTH
Actinnomyces bovis ....
.... *Actinomyces bovis*
actiontherapy .... actinotherapy
activ imunity .... active immunity
activsite .... active site
acttinomycosis .... actinomycosis
acttive transport ...... active transport
aculocardiac reflex ....
.... oculocardiac reflex
Acutane .... Accutane
acwired .... acquired
acyupuncture .... acupuncture
acyute brain disorders ....
.... acute brain disorders
adanine .... adenine
adanoids .... adenoids
adapose .... adipose
adative .... additive**
Addam's apple .... Adam's apple
addaptation .... adaptation
addenitis .... adenitis
addeno- (pre) .... adeno-
addenoma .... adenoma
addenoseen triphosphate ....
..... adenosine triphosphate (ATP)
addherent .... adherent
addhesive compress ....
.... adhesive compress
addick .... addict

3

Incorrect	Correct	Incorrect	Correct
addiktive	**addictive**	aferant	**afferent****
addiology	**audiology**	aferent pathway	**afferent pathway**
addip- (pre)	**adip-**	affebrile	**afebrile**
addipic asid	**adipic acid**	affektive slumber	**affective slumber**
addipo- (pre)	**adipo-**	afliction	**affliction**
addipocyte	**adipocyte**	afluema	**affluemna**
Addler	**Adler**	afluent	**affluent****
addnexa	**adnexa**	afotericin	**amphotericin**
addrenal cortical hyperfunction	**adrenal cortical hyperfunction**	afradisiac	**aphrodisiac****
addreniline	**adrenalin**	afrent neuron	**afferent neuron**
addrenocorticotropic hormone	**adrenocorticotropic hormone**	aftabirth	**afterbirth**
addsorb	**adsorb****	agaranulocitosis	**agranulocytosis**
addult	**adult**	ager	**agger****
addverse event	**adverse event**	aggar	**agar****
adennocarsinoma	**adenocarcinoma**	agglootinin	**agglutinin**
adennosine	**adenosine**	aggnosia	**agnosia**
adernergic	**adrenergic**	aggonal	**agonal**
adgita	**agita**	aggranular endoplasmic reticulum	**agranular endoplasmic reticulum**
adh	**ADH**	aggraphia	**agraphia**
adheesion	**adhesion**	aggresive	**aggressive**
adhisive tape	**adhesive tape**	aggue	**ague**
adick	**addict**	aginist	**agonist**
adiction	**addiction**	aglutination	**agglutination**
adinnexitis	**adnexitis**	agrannalocytes	**agranulocytes**
adinosine diphosphate	**adenosine diphosphate**	agression	**aggression**
adinoydo- (pre)	**adenoido-**	AIDDS victim	**AIDS victim**
Adison's disease	**Addison's disease**	AIDES	**AIDS****
aditive	**additive****	AIDZ-related complex	**AIDS-related complex**
aditive-free	**additive-free**	airobics	**aerobics**
Adlirien psychotherapy	**Adlerian psychotherapy**	airofagia	**aerophagia**
adneksa uteri	**adnexa uteri**	airosell	**aerocele****
adp	**ADP**	airotherapy	**aerotherapy**
adreenal gland	**adrenal gland**	ajavant therapy	**adjuvant therapy**
adrenatrofin	**adrenotrophin**	ajunctive chemotherapy	**adjunctive chemotherapy**
adrennal hypofunction	**adrenal hypofunction**	akapneal	**acapnial****
adrennosterone	**adrenosterone**	akathexis	**acathexis****
aduct	**adduct**	akcident	**accident**
aductor	**adductor****	akne	**acne**
aersickness	**airsickness**	akonite	**aconite**
aertitis	**aortitis**	akorea	**acorea****
afasia	**aphasia****	akoustic nerve	**acoustic nerve**
afect	**affect****	akr- (pre)	**acr-**

4

Incorrect	Correct	Incorrect	Correct
akramegaly	acromegaly	All-Anon	Al-Anon**
akrid	acrid**	allapath	allopath**
akro- (pre)	acro-	allbinism	albinism
akrondoplasia	achondroplasia	allbumen	albumen**
aksial	axial	allbumin	albumin**
aktin	actin	allcohol	alcohol
akting out	acting out	alldose	aldose
aktinomycine	actinomycin	Allexander technique	
aktive birth	active birth		Alexander technique
akupressure	acupressure	allexia	alexia
akute	acute	allgo- (pre)	algo-
akwa-erobics	aqua-aerobics	alliment	aliment**
akweous liquor	aqueous liquor	allimentotherapy	alimentotherapy
akwuired imune deficiency		Allka-Seltzer	Alka Seltzer
sindrome		allopecia	alopecia
	acquired immune deficiency syndrome	allpha rhythm	alpha rhythm
akyute abdomen	acute abdomen	allternative medicine	
al- (pre)	all-		alternative medicine
alabido	alibido	alltitude sickness	altitude sickness
alagraft	allograft	alltrose	altrose
alamentary canal	alimentary canal	allveolo- (pre)	alveolo-
Alan-Doisy hormone		Allzheimer's disease	
	Allen-Doisy hormone		Alzheimer's disease
Alargan	Allergan**	alo- (pre)	allo-
albimunuria	albuminuria	alopathy	allopathy**
albyoomin- (pre)	albumin-**	alose	aloes
albyumino- (pre)	albumino-	alosome	allosome
albyuminoid	albuminoid	alosteric enzyme	allosteric enzyme
alcaholism	alcoholism	alpha-phetoprotein	
alcalosis	alkalosis		alpha-fetoprotein
aldusterone	aldosterone	alpher wave	alpha wave
aleanation	alienation	Alsheimer's disease	
alectramyogram	electromyogram**		Alzheimer's disease
alegenic	allogenic	alurgist	allergist
alegy	allergy	alvaolus	alveolus
alele	allele	alveelar pressure	alveolar pressure
alement	ailment**	alviolar bone	alveolar bone
alementary	alimentary**	alvyolar ventilation	
alfa cells	alpha cells		alveolar ventilation
alfar-amylase	alpha-amylase	ama	AMA
-algea (suff)	-algia	amabarbital sodium	
alinine	alanine**		amobarbital sodium
Alkoholics Anonimous		amadase	amidase
	Alcoholics Anonymous	amadeen	amidine**
allajen	allergen**	amalase	amylase
allamentery	alimentary**	amanestic syndrome	
			amnestic syndrome

5

Incorrect	Correct	Incorrect	Correct

amanopolypeptidase ....
.... **aminopolypeptidase**
amarosis .... **amaurosis**
ambleo- (pre) .... **amblyo-**
ambyalance .... **ambulance**
ambyulatory .... **ambulatory**
ameebiasis .... **amebiasis**
amenia.............................. **anemia**
ameocentesis .... **amniocentesis**
amfetamine sulfate ....
.... **amphetamine sulfate**
amilopsin .... **amylopsin**
aminnopyrine .... **aminopyrin****
aminoinfusion .... **amnioinfusion**
Amital .... **Amytal**
ammandin .... **amandin**
ammbavert .... **ambivert**
ammblyopia .... **amblyopia**
ammeba................ **ameba** or **amoeba**
ammenorea .... **amenorrhea**
ammentia .... **amentia**
Ammerican Medical Association ....
.... **American Medical Association**
ammidin .... **amidin****
ammino acid .... **amino acid**
ammiotensin .... **amniotensin**
ammobarbital .... **amobarbital**
ammonneum chloride ....
.... **ammonium chloride**
ammorfus .... **amorphous****
ammoxicillin .... **amoxicillin**
ammpicillin .... **ampicillin**
ammyl- (pre) .... **amyl-**
ammyl nitrite .... **amyl nitrite**
ammylo- (pre) .... **amylo-**
ammylopectin .... **amylopectin**
ammyotrophic lateral sclerosis ......
.... **amyotrophic lateral sclerosis**
anmion .... **amnion**
amnisia............................ **amnesia**
amnopeptidase .... **aminopeptidase**
amny- (pre) .... **amni-**
amnyo- (pre) .... **amnio-**
amnyotin .... **Amniotin**
amonia .... **ammonia**
amorefuss...................... **amorphus****
ampit .... **armpit**
ampyule .... **ampule****

amybic dysentery ... **amebic dysentery**
amytripyline .... **amitriptyline**
anabbolism .... **anabolism**
anacastic personality ....
.... **anancastic** or **anakastic**
personality
anadyne .... **anodyne**
anafylaxis .... **anaphylaxis**
analisis .... **analysis****
anama .... **anima****
anamolous .... **anomalous**
anarectal disorders ....
.... **anorectal disorders**
anarobic .... **anaerobic**
anastheeseeoligist ..... **anesthesiologist**
anasthesiology .... **anesthesiology**
and-dyastolic volume ....
.... **end-diastolic volume**
anderosterone .... **androsterone**
anditoksin .... **antitoxin**
androginous .... **androgynous****
androjenous............... **androgenous****
aneclisiss .... **anaclisis****
anelgesic .... **analgesic**
anemy .... **anomie****
anessthetic .... **anesthetic**
anfotericin .... **amphotericin**
angery macrophage ....
.... **angary macrophage**
angore .... **angor****
angsiety .... **anxiety**
angur .... **anger****
angyocardiography ....
.... **angiocardiography**
anhidro- (pre) .... **anhydro-**
anibolic steroid .... **anabolic steroid**
anicusis .... **anacusis**
anisthyl .... **anysthyl**
anjeeoma .... **angioma**
anjeplasty .... **angioplasty**
anji- (pre) .... **angi-**
anjina .... **angina**
anjio- (pre) .... **angio-**
anjioma .... **angioma**
ankel .... **ankle**
anksiety neurosis ..... **anxiety neurosis**
ankyl/o- (pre) .... **anchyl/o-**
ann- (pre) .... **an-**

anna- (pre) .... ana-
annabolic steroid hormones ....
.... anabolic steroid hormones
annabolism .... anabolism
Annacin .... Anacin
annaclassis .... anaclasis**
annafase .... anaphase
annalgesia .... analgesia
annalogues .... analogues
annal personality ..... anal personality
annalytic psychology ....
.... analytic psychology
annatomy .... anatomy
anncylosis .... ankylosis
anndrogen .... androgen
annencefaly .... anencephaly
annerexia nervous ....
.... anorexia nervosa
annesthesia .... anesthesia
anngina pectoris .... angina pectoris
anngiography .... angiography
annimality .... animality
anniography .... amniography
annlage .... anlage
anno- (pre) .... ano-
annomalies .... anomalies
annorkous .... anorchous**
annovulation .... anovulation
annoxia .... anoxia
anntaginism .... antagonism
annte- (pre) .... ante-
anntebody-positive ....
.... antibody positive
anntelmintic .... anthelmintic
annterior chamber ... anterior chamber
annth- (pre) .... anth-
annthelmintic .... anthelmintic
annthraks .... anthrax
anntibody seropositivity ....
.... antibody seropositivity
anntimicin A .... antimicin A
anntipuritic .... antipruritic
anntispazmodic .... antispasmodic
anntrum .... antrum
anomium carbonate ....
.... ammonium carbonate
anooploidy .... aneuploidy
anorecus .... anorchus**

anphetamine .... amphetamine
anputation .... amputation
antabody-negative ....
.... antibody negative
antaceptic .... antiseptic
antadote .... antidote**
antaggonist .... antagonist
antajen .... antigen
antapirene .... antipyrine
ante-arhythmic .... antiarrhythmic
antearior .... anterior
antebiotic .... antibiotic
antebody seronegativity ....
.... antibody seronegativity
anteclotting .... anticlotting
ante-coagulent .... anticoagulant
ante-convulsant .... anticonvulsant
antedyuretic hormone ....
.... antidiuretic hormone
antee .... anti**
anteflatulent .... antiflatulent
antefunjal .... antifungal
ante-histamine .... antihistamine
antekolinergic .... anticholinergic
antemeer .... antimere**
antemer .... antimer**
anteprosstagladinsisobutyl
nitrate ....
.... antiprostaglandinsisobutyl
nitrate
antepyritic .... antipyretic
ante-seerum .... antiserum
anteshok trousers ....
.... antishock trousers
antesocial personality ....
.... antisocial personality
antesychotics .... antipsychotics
antevinin .... antivenin
ante-virus .... antivirus
antiacid .... antacid
Antibuse .... Antabuse
anti-dipressant .... antidepressant
antiediaretic .... antidiuretic
antie-inflammatory ....
.... anti-inflammatory
antiflexion .... anteflexion
antigrade .... antegrade
antimetic .... antiemetic

Incorrect	Correct
antimortim	**antemortem**
antinatil	**antenatel**
antipartim	**antepartum**
antirior	**anterior**
antisipation	**anticipation**
anty	**anti-**
antyangsiety drugs	**antianxiety drug**
antybody	**antibody**
antymikrobial	**antimicrobial**
antyoksident	**antioxidant**
antysoshial personality	**antisocial personality**
antytusive	**antitussive**
anumus	**animus****
anxeity reaction	**anxiety reaction**
anxyety disorder	**anxiety disorder**
anyulary	**annulary**
anyurism	**aneurism**
aorrtic arch	**aortic arch**
aorter	**aorta**
aorrticbody chemoreceptor	**aortic-body chemoreceptor**
apaplexy	**apoplexy**
apattite supressant	**appetite suppressant**
apendectomy	**appendectomy**
apendics	**appendix**
apendiko- (pre)	**appendico-**
apendo- (pre)	**appendo-**
apenzyme	**apoenzyme**
apetite	**appetite****
apicrine	**apocrine**
aplacation	**application**
aplasstic anemia	**aplastic anemia**
aplide psychology	**applied psychology**
appatite	**apatite****
appenndisitis	**appendicitis**
appex	**apex**
appgar score	**Apgar score**
appnea	**apnea**
appocrine secretion	**apocrine secretion**
apposing margins	**opposing margins**

Incorrect	Correct
appothacery	**apothecary**
apracksia	**apraxia**
apsorbtion	**absorption**
aramatic spirits of amonia	**aromatic spirits of ammonia**
arasole	**aerosol****
arbanose	**arabinose**
arborvirus	**arbovirus**
arc	**ARC**
arck	**arc**
arcyuate	**arcuate**
are hunger	**air hunger**
Areomycin	**Aureomycin**
Argarol	**Argyrol**
argenine	**arginine**
ariban	**araban****
arinavirus	**arenavirus**
arjinase	**arginase**
arkeye	**arc-eye**
arktype	**archetyper**
aro- (pre)	**aero-**
arobic	**aerobic**
aroembolism	**aeroembolism**
arojenous	**aerogenous****
arosole therapy	**aerosol therapy**
arouzel	**arousal**
arraknoid villus	**arachnoid villus**
arrcuate vessels	**arcuate vessels**
arribin	**arabin****
arricle	**auricle**
arrmamentarium	**armamentarium**
arrnica	**arnica**
arroma-therapy	**aromatherapy**
arrotherapeutics	**aerotherapeutics**
arrsenic	**arsenic**
arrteriolo- (pre)	**arteriolo-**
arrthro- (pre)	**arthro-**
arrtifishial insemination	**artificial insemination**
arsinotherapy	**arsenotherapy**
artafficial lung	**artificial lung**
artaficial heart	**artificial heart**
artefishal	**artificial**
arterreolar resistance	**arteriolar resistance**
arterriol	**arteriole**

arterry .... **artery**
arthero- (pre) .... **athero-**
artheroma .... **atheroma**
arthrascope .... **arthroscope**
artifficial limb .... **artificial limb**
artireal baroreceptors ....
.... **arterial baroreceptors**
artirio- (pre) .... **arterio-**
artiriosklerosis .... **arteriosclerosis**
arttificial kidney ...... **artificial kidney**
arythmia ....
..... **arhythmia** or arrhythmia****
asadosis .... **acidosis**
asazerine .... **azaserine**
aseetil .... **acetyl****
asefalic .... **acephalic**
A sells .... **A cells**
ASE mixture .... **ACE mixture**
asentric .... **acentric**
asessment .... **assessment**
asetabulum .... **acetabulum**
asetaminophen .... **acetaminophen**
asetanilide .... **acetanilide**
asetic .... **acetic**
asetilcholine .... **acetylcholine**
asettylsalicylic acid ....
.... **acetylsalicylic acid**
asfixiation .... **asphyxiation**
asiclovir .... **acyclovir**
asid-fast bacteria .... **acid-fast bacteria**
asimilation .... **assimilation**
asimptomatic .... **asymptomatic**
askorbic acid .... **ascorbic acid**
asma .... **asthma**
asperater .... **aspirator**
asperin .... **aspirin**
assbestose .... **asbestos****
assending colon .... **ascending colon**
assepsis .... **asepsis**
assetophenetidin .... **acetophenetidin**
assid .... **acid****
assinus .... **acinus**
assitia .... **asitia**
asspartic acid .... **aspartic acid**
asspect .... **aspect**
asspiration .... **aspiration**

assthenic reaction ... **asthenic reaction**
asstigmatism .... **astigmatism**
asstringent .... **astringent**
assylum .... **asylum**
assymtomaticity ...... **asymptomaticity**
astrogeloid .... **astragaloid**
asyclic .... **acyclic**
atendant .... **attendant**
atendding .... **attending**
atendyuated virus .... **attenuated virus**
athalete's foot .... **athlete's foot**
atheerosklerosis .... **atherosclerosis**
athritis .... **arthritis****
athroscopy .... **arthroscopy**
ativism .... **atavism**
atp .... **ATP**
atraphy .... **atrophy**
atripine .... **atropine**
atrition .... **attrition**
attabrine .... **Atabrine**
attaxia .... **ataxia**
attelo- (pre) .... **atelo-**
attennding physician ....
.... **attending physician**
attlas .... **atlas**
attom .... **atom**
attony .... **atony**
attopy .... **atopy**
attresia .... **atresia**
audeometer .... **audiometer**
aunt- (pre) .... **ant-**
aunterior lobe disorders ....
.... **anterior lobe disorder**
aunti- (pre) .... **anti-**
aural thermometer **oral thermometer**
autaclaving .... **autoclaving**
autagraph .... **autograft**
autamaticity .... **automaticity**
autamiton .... **automaton****
autasom .... **autosome**
auterregulation .... **autoregulation**
autimmune disease ....
.... **autoimmune disease**
autisomal recessive ....
.... **autosomal recessive**
autommatin .... **automatin****

Incorrect	Correct
autommune	**autoimmune**
automonic	**autonomic**
auttologous	**autologous**
auttoserum therapy	**autoserum therapy**
auxillary	**axillary****
aviolus	**alveolus**
avoident pursonality	**avoidant personality**
avoydance reaction	**avoidance reaction**
avrage length of stay	**average length of stay**
avursion therapy	**aversion therapy**
Avvertin	**Avertin**
avvulsion	**avulsion** or **evulsion**
awbicular	**orbicular**
awbicularis	**orbicularis**
awdative	**auditive****
awdiogram	**audiogram**
awditory sells	**auditory cells**
awganism	**organism**
awgmentation mammoplasty	**augmentation mammoplasty**
awl-or-none response	**all** or **none response**
awra	**aura****
awrbittal	**orbital****
awrganically	**organically**
awriginal	**original**
awrphan	**orphan**
awrthopnea	**orthopnea**
awscultation	**auscultation**
awthoscope	**orthoscope**

Incorrect	Correct
awtism	**autism**
awtoclave	**autoclave**
awtogenic training	**autogenic training**
awtomation	**automation****
awtopsy	**autopsy**
axalary dissection	**axillary dissection**
axalery hair	**axillary hair**
axidently	**accidentally**
axidothimadine	**azidothymadine**
axxila	**axilla**
axxis	**axis**
axxojenous	**axogenous****
axxon	**axon**** or **axone****
axxon transport	**axon transport**
Ayce bandage	**ACE bandage**
aycoria	**acoria****
AYDS	**AIDS****
AYDS test	**AIDS test**
ayebrow	**eyebrow**
ayerophagia	**aerophagia**
ayling	**ailing**
aynus	**anus****
ayort- (pre)	**aort-**
ayortic valve disease	**aortic valve disease**
ayorto- (pre)	**aorto-**
ayseksual	**asexual**
aytrium	**atrium**
azbestosis	**asbestosis****
azospermia	**azoospermia**
azt	**AZT**

B

Incorrect	Correct
Babbinsky	**Babinski**
babby-batering	**baby-battering**
bac	**BAC**
bacatracin	**bacitracin**
bacbone	**backbone**
baccteri- (pre)	**bacteri-**
baccteria	**bacteria**
back-aik	**backache**
backteremia	**bacteremia**

Incorrect	Correct
backterial therapy	**bacterial therapy**
back-up hospitel	**backup hospital**
bacteriel	**bacterial**
bacteriel endocarditis	**bacterial endocarditis**
bacterreology	**bacteriology**
bacterrotherepy	**bacteriotherapy**
bacteryostat	**bacteriostat**

Incorrect	Correct
bactirium	**bacterium**
bactoricide	**bactericide****
bactrolysins	**bacteriolysins**
bad breth	**bad breath**
baff	**bath****
baise	**base**
baiter blocker	**beta blocker**
baiter wave	**beta wave**
bak	**back**
bakeing soda	**baking soda**
baktirea	**bacteria**
balence	**balance****
balinitis	**balanitis**
balland-socket joint	
	ball-and-socket joint
balledness	**baldness**
ballsam	**balsam**
ballune	**balloon**
baloon angioplasty	
	balloon angioplasty
balotement	**ballottement**
bambu sugar	**bamboo sugar**
bammboo spine	**bamboo spine**
bam of Gilead	**balm of Gilead**
bandade	**Band Aid**
bandige	**bandage**
bangg	**bhang**
banned-aid sterilization	
	band-aid sterilization
bannting	**Banting**
barbaturic acid	**barbituric acid**
barbichurate	**barbiturate**
Barbody	**Barr body**
baren	**barren**
bariam sulfate	**barium sulfate**
barier contraceptives	
	barrier contraceptives
barm	**balm****
barr	**bar****
barrbital	**barbital**
barric	**baric**
barrium enema	**barium enema**
barrley sugar	**barley sugar**
Barrlow's syndrome	
	Barlow's syndrome
barroreceptor	**baroreceptor**
Barrtholin glands	**Bartholin glands**
Barrton bandage	**Barton bandage**

Incorrect	Correct
baryum meal	**barium meal**
bassal	**basal****
basel body temperature method	
.. **basal body temperature method**	
Basel Nomica Anatomica	
	Basle Nomina Anatomica
basil metabolism	**basal metabolism**
basili	**bacilli**
basill- (pre)	**bacill-**
basillary dysentery	
	bacillary dysentery
basillus	**bacillus**
bassal ganglia	**basal ganglia**
bassess	**bases****
bassic	**basic**
bata blocker	**beta blocker**
bater	**batter**
bater wave	**beta wave**
battel fatigue	**battle fatigue**
baul	**ball****
bawrn	**born****
baysal metabolic rate	
	basal metabolic rate
baysis	**basis****
baysment membrane	
	basement membrane
bayta	**beta****
baythe	**bathe****
bazal	**basal****
bazel-cell carcinoma	
	basal-cell carcinoma
bazophil	**basophil**
bearth	**berth****
beat sugar	**beet sugar**
bedd occupancy	**bed occupancy**
bed-pann	**bedpan**
bedrest	**bed rest**
bedriden	**bedridden**
bed-side manor	**bedside manner**
bedsoar	**bedsore**
bed weting	**bedwetting**
Bee cell	**B cell**
beehavior therapy	
	behavior therapy
beehavioral medicine	
	behavioral medicine
beestiality	**bestiality**
behavierism	**behaviorism**

11

Incorrect	Correct	Incorrect	Correct
behayvior	behavior	binay	Binet
beladona	belladonna	bindeing site	binding site
bele	bel**	bineder boric acid	
bellch	belch		binder boric acid
Belle	Bell**	binign orgasmic headaches	
bell indifference	belle indifference		benign orgasmic headaches
belly butten	bellybutton	binje-purje syndrome	
Bel's palsy	Bell's palsy		binge-purge syndrome
bely	belly**	bioefeedback	biofeedback
benine	benign	bioessay	bioassay
bens	bends	bioppsy	biopsy
bensacaine	benzocaine	biosinthesis	biosynthesis
benzedrine	Benzadrine	biotek	biotech**
benzoine	benzoin**	bio-teknology	biotechnology
bern	burn	biottin	biotin
berry-berry	beriberi	bippolar disorder	bipolar disorder
bersa	bursa	biseps	biceps
bersitis	bursitis	bisinosis	byssinosis
berso- (pre)	burso-	bisstory	bistoury
berth canal	birth canal	bittwing radiograph	
berth-kontrol pill	birth control pill		bite-wing radiograph
berth mark	birthmark	bizmuth	bismuth
berybery	beriberi	blaceye	black eye
beter	better**	blackheds	blackheads
betta	beta**	black owt	blackout**
betta cells	beta cells	blaclung	black lung
bettaramylase	beta-amylase	blacwatter fever	blackwater fever
better rhythm	beta rhythm	bladdor	bladder
beutirophenones	butyrophenone	blader augmentation	
bial duct	bile duct		bladder augmentation
biassay	bioassay	blak-and-blue mark	
bibbliotherapy	bibliotherapy		black-and-blue mark
bickloride of mercury		blakout	black out**
	bichloride of mercury	blanc-state hypothesis	
bidday	bidet		blank-state hypothesis
bikloride of mercury		-blassed (suff)	-blast
	bichloride of mercury	blasst- (pre)	blast-
bikuspid	bicuspid	blassto- (pre)	blasto-
Bilig exercises	Billig exercises	*Blasstomyces braziliensis*	
Bilings method	Billings method		*Blastomyces brasiliensis*
bille salts	bile salts	blastamykosis	blastomycosis
billi- (pre)	bili-	blebb	bleb
billiary colic	biliary colic	bleder	bleeder
billirubin	bilirubin	bleeching powder	bleaching powder
billyrubinemia	bilirubinemia	blefar- (pre)	blephar-
bilogics	biologics	blefaritis	blepharitis
bilyous	bilious	blefaro- (pre)	blepharo-

Incorrect	Correct
blefferoplasty	blepharoplasty
blenorhagia	blennorrhagia
blew ointment	blue ointment
b limphocyte	B lymphocyte
blineness	blindness
bliomicin	bleomycin
blisster	blister
Blocc	Blocq**
bloc grants	block grants
blod alkohol concentration	blood alcohol concentration
bloe	blow
Blok	Bloch**
blok	block**
bloking	blocking
bloking antibody	blocking antibody
blokk	block**
blokker	blocker
bloodbank	blood bank
blood-brane barrier	blood-brain barrier
blood-clott	blood clot
blood-componant	blood component
blood-cownt	blood count
blooddoner	blood donor
blood grupe	blood group
bloodleting	bloodletting
blood mobil	bloodmobile
blood poysening	blood poisoning
blood-presher couff	blood pressure cuff
bloodpreshur	blood pressure
blood-shuger	blood sugar
bloodstreem	bloodstream
blood tipes	blood types
bloodtiping	blood typing
blood yurea nitrogen	blood urea nitrogen
blotsh	blotch
blubaby	blue baby
blud	blood
blud-alcohol content	blood alcohol content
bluddy flucks	bloody flux
blue cross	Blue Cross
Blue Sheeld	Blue Shield
blured vision	blurred vision

Incorrect	Correct
bmr	BMR
b'nai	Binet
boan	bone
boarderline personality	borderline personality
boddy	body
boddy-building	bodybuilding
body-flooids	body fluids
body-kontouring	body contouring
body-langwage	body language
body mecanics	body mechanics
bodyrap	body wrap
body-skanner	body scanner
body-skeema	body schema
bollus	bolus
bomb of Gilead	balm of Gilead
boney	bony
bon graft	bone graft
bonned	bond
booba	bouba
booboo	bubo**
boogie	bougie
boosom	bosom
boosster shot	booster shot
bord certified physician	board certified physician
bordeline	borderline
border baby	boarder baby
borditela	*Bordetella*
borelia	*Borelia* or *Borrelia*
Bornehome disease	Bornholm disease
borrax	borax
borrborigmus	borborygmus
borric acid	boric acid
borrn	borne**
Borroughs-Wellcome	Burroughs-Wellcome
bos	boss
bottulin	botulin
botyulism	botulism
bowl evacuant	bowel evacuant
bowwel	bowel**
boyl	boil
brachie- (pre)	brachy-
bracial	brachial
braddykinin	bradykinin

13

Incorrect	Correct
bradicardia	bradycardia
braine-damage	brain damage
brakeout	break out**
brake-thru bleeding ...... breakthrough bleeding	
brakewind	break wind
brakial nerve	brachial nerve
branestem	brain stem
brase	brace
brawd-spectrum	broad-spectrum
brayces	braces
braydy- (pre)	brady-
brayk	break**
brayn	brain
breach presintation ...... breech presentation	
breakthroogh bleeding ...... breakthrough bleeding	
breast awgmentation ...... breast augmentation	
breast bone	breastbone
breastfeed	breast-feed
breething	breathing
Breoski	Brioschi
bresbone	breastbone
bresst tosis	breast ptosis
brest	breast
brest-reduction	breast reduction
brethalyzer	Breathalyzer
brethlessness	breathlessness
brige	bridge
Brisstol-Meyers Squibb ...... Bristol-Myers Squibb	
Brite	Bright**
brite	bright**
Brites disease	Bright's disease
brittish gum	British gum
broche	broach
broemin	bromine
bromied	bromide
brommidrossis	bromidrosis
bromoe seltzer	Bromo Seltzer
bronkadilator	bronchodilator
bronkascope	bronchoscope
bronki- (pre)	bronchi-
bronkial asma	bronchial asthma
bronkio- (pre)	bronchio-
bronkiss	bronchus

Incorrect	Correct
bronkitus	bronchitis
bronkyole	bronchiole**
bronnch- (pre)	bronch-
bronnchospazm	bronchospasm
brooser	bruiser
broot	bruit
brounlung	brown lung
brouw	brow
bruecelosis	brucellosis
bruksism	bruxism
bruse	bruise
brusella	brucella
buckle cavity	buccal cavity
buco- (pre)	bucco-
buctooth	bucktooth
Bud	Budd**
budd	bud**
bufer therapy	buffer therapy
bufferd asprin	buffered aspirin
buffrin	Bufferin
bula	bulla
bulbuss	bulbus**
bulc floe	bulk flow
bullb sirynge	bulb syringe
bullbus	bulbous**
bullimia	bulimia
bun	BUN
bunp	bump
bunyon	bunion
burn-owt	burnout
Burros solution	Burow's solution
burth	birth**
burth defect	birth defect
buticaine sulfate	butacaine sulfate
butil	butyl
buttox	buttocks
buttz	butts**
butz	buts**
by- (pre)	bi-
byamedicine	biomedicine
bycarbonate of soda ...... bicarbonate of soda	
bycuspid	bicuspid
byel salts	bile salts
byepass	bypass
byfokal	bifocal
byfurcation	bifurcation
byillogical clock	biological clock

Incorrect	Correct	Incorrect	Correct
byle	bile**	byonics	bionics
byoassay	bioassay	byotherapy	biotherapy
byoenergetics	bioenergetics	byubonic plague	bubonic plague
byoethics	bioethics	byutacaine	butacaine
byoluminesence	bioluminescence		

C

Incorrect	Correct	Incorrect	Correct
cacco- (pre)	caco-	cappallary	capillary
caccodontia	cacodontia	capplet	caplet**
cachment aria	catchment area	cappsid	capsid
caddaver	cadaver	capsyule	capsule**
caf	calf	carbahidrate	carbohydrate
cafeene	caffeine	carddiomeopathy	cardiomyopathy
cain sugar	cane sugar	carde- (pre)	cardi-
calabrate	calibrate	cardeac stenosis	cardiac stenosis
calasthenics	calisthenics	cardeo- (pre)	cardio-
calcyalus	calculus**	cardeo salsa	Cardio salsa
calimine lotion	calamine lotion	cardiak massage	cardiac massage
calis	callous**	cardiaresperatory endurance	
calkaneus	calcaneus		cardiorespiratory endurance
calkulous	calculous**	cardipullmonary resussitation	
callc- (pre)	calc-		cardiopulmonary resuscitation
callcitonin	calcitonin	cardiscope	cardioscope
callcium carbonate		cardiyografy	cardiography
	calcium carbonate	-cardya (suff)	-cardia**
callender method	calendar method	cardyac output	cardiac output
callor	calor**	carees	caries**
calose	callose**	carese	carries**
calsi- (pre)	calci-	carinary artery disease	
calsinosis	calcinosis		coronary artery disease
calsium channel blocker		carnatin	carnitine
	calcium channel blocker	carrbimycin	carbomycin
camfer	camphor**	carrbolic acid	carbolic acid
camodulin	calmodulin	carrbonic anhydrase	
C amp	cAMP		carbonic anhydrase
campilobactor	Campylobacter	carrdiac hormone	cardiac hormone
camra	camera	carrdioligy	cardiology
cancre	canker**	carrer	carer**
candiasis	candidiasis	carroteen	carotene
candidda	Candida**	carrotid artery	carotid artery
canibis	cannabis	carrpall tunnel syndrome	
cannal	canal		carpal tunnel syndrome
canndida	Candida**	carrsinogen	carcinogen
canser	cancer**	carryer	carrier**
canyulation	cannulation	carsanoma	carcinoma
capatate	capitate**	car sickness	carsickness

Incorrect	Correct
carsino- (pre)	carcino-
cashay	cachet
casheksia	cachexia
casin	casein
casolet	cassolette
casskara sagrada	cascara sagrada
casster oil	castor oil
casstration	castration
cathasis	catharsis
cathitter	catheter
Cathollicon	catholicon
catistrofic coverage	catastrophic coverage
catt- (pre)	cat-
catta- (pre)	cata-
cattabolism	catabolism
cattakolamines	catecholamines
cattanemia	catamenia
cattar	catarrh
catteract	cataract
cattitonia	catatonia
catt scan	CAT scan
cattscratch disease	cat-scratch disease
caull	caul**
causstic	caustic
cavvernus	cavernous
cavvum	cavum
cawd- (pre)	caud-
cawda eckwina	cauda equina
cawdo- (pre)	caudo-
cawgh syrup	cough syrup
cawl	call**
cawpse	corpse**
cawre	core**
cawsal agent	causal agent
cawterise	cauterize
cayne sugar	cane sugar
cayrgiver	care-giver
cayse history	case history
caysson disease	caisson disease
cebum	sebum
ceckum	cecum
cedation	sedation
ceecal	cecal
ceed graft	seed graft
ceel	seal**
Cee-section	C-section

Incorrect	Correct
cefalalgia	cephalgia or cephalalgia
cefaloridine	cephaloridine
cel divison	cell division
-celle (suff)	-cell
cellective arteriography	selective arteriography
cell meediated immunity	cell-mediated immunity
celobiose	cellobiose
celyallose	cellulose
celyulitus	cellulitis
cemeiotics	semeiotics or semiotics
cemenmtim	cementum
cemiotics	semeiotics or semiotics
cenile dementia	senile dementia
cenilis	senilis
cenntral hearing loss	central hearing loss
cenntrefuge	centrifuge
censation	sensation
censer	censor**
censibility	sensibility
censitivity	sensitivity
censitization	sensitization
centeral thermoreceptors	central thermoreceptors
centinal polip	sentinel polyp
cepperating saw	separating saw
ceppsis	sepsis
ceptal deviation	septal deviation
ceptic	septic
cepticemia	septicemia
cepticemic meningitis	septicemic meningitis
ceptum	septum
cer- (pre)	ser-
cerbral aqueduct	cerebral aqueduct
cercle	circle
cercomstans	circumstance
cerculatory system	circulatory system
cereebrospinal sistem	cerebrospinal system
cerees	series
cerface	surface
cero- (pre)	sero-
cerologic	serologic
cerological	serological

16

cerological tests .... **serological tests**
cerology .... **serology**
ceromuscular .... **seromuscular**
ceronegativity .... **seronegativity**
ceropositivity .... **seropositivity**
ceropurulent discharge ....
.... **seropurulent discharge**
cerosal .... **serosal**
cerotherapy .... **serotherapy**
cerotonin .... **serotinin**
cerrated .... **cerated****
cerrebellum .... **cerebellum****
cerrebro- (pre) .... **cerebro-**
cerreous............................ **cereous****
cerribral palsy .... **cerebral palsy**
cerrous .... **cerous****
cerrum-cholesterol ....
.... **serum-cholesterol**
cerrumenolytic .... **cerumenolytic**
cerrvical dysplasia ....
.... **cervical dysplasia**
cerrvikal-mucus method ....
.... **cervical-mucus method**
cerrvix............................ **cervix**
cerum .... **serum**
cervacal incompetence ....
.... **cervical incompetence**
cervasectomy .... **cervicectomy**
cervature of the spine ....
.... **curvature of the spine**
cervay .... **survey**
cervecal ose .... **cervical os**
cervisitis .... **cervicitis**
cerviss .... **service**
cervival .... **survival**
cession .... **session**
ceverance .... **severance**
cevere............................ **severe**
cevered tendin .... **severed tendon**
ceverity .... **severity**
ceytoxin .... **cytoxin**
Chain-Stokes respiration ....
.... **Cheyne-Stokes respiration**
chanel............................ **channel**
chaning .... **chaining**
chankroid .... **chancroid**
channge of life............ **change of life**
chaping .... **chapping**

charcott .... **Charcot**
charege nerse .... **charge nurse**
charkos joint .... **Charcot's joint**
Charly horse .... **charley horse**
charrity patient .... **charity patient**
cheak...................................... **cheek**
cheeck bone .... **cheekbone**
cheef cells .... **chief cells**
cheemotherapy .... **chemotherapy**
cheif resident .... **chief resident**
chekup....................................**checkup**
chellating agents ...... **chelating agents**
chemareceptors .... **chemoreceptors**
chemecal specificity ....
.... **chemical specificity**
chemm- (pre) .... **chem-**
chemmi- (pre) .... **chemi-**
chemmical peel .... **chemical peel**
chemmical sence .... **chemical sense**
chemmist................................. **chemist**
chemmo- (pre) .... **chemo-**
chemmoresistance .... **chemoresistance**
chemmo-taxes .... **chemotaxis**
chemmotherapy .... **chemotherapy**
chessed x-ray .... **chest x-ray**
chesst .... **chest**
chieropractic adjustment ....
.... **chiropractic adjustment**
chigella .... **shigella**
chiken-pox .... **chickenpox**
childe .... **child**
chile-development ....
.... **child development**
chiled abuse .... **child abuse**
chillblane .... **chilblain**
chilldern's hospital ....
.... **children's hospital**
chilled bed fever .... **childbed fever**
chillo- (pre) .... **chilo-**
chilosis .... **cheilosis**
chime .... **chyme**
chinn .... **chin**
chipp .... **chip**
chlawpromizine .... **chlorpromazine**
chlawramine .... **chloramine**
chloremphenicol ..... **chloramphenicol**
chloremycetin .... **Chloromycetin**
chlorrine of lime .... **chlorine of lime**

chlorrtettracycline ... **chlortetracycline**
choak .... **choke**
choalelithiasis .... **cholelithiasis**
choclit .... **chocolate**
chokeing .... **choking**
choll- (pre) .... **chol-**
chollangia .... **cholangia**
cholle- (pre) .... **chole-**
chollecyst .... **cholecyst**
chollo- (pre) .... **cholo-**
chollosistitis .... **cholecystitis****
choral .... **chloral**
chorroid plexus .... **choroid plexus**
chorryonic gonadotropin ....
.... **chorionic gonadotropin**
chrommaprotein .... **chromaprotein**
chronnic fatigue syndrome ....
.... **chronic fatigue syndrome**
chyl- (pre) .... **cheil-**
chylitis .... **cheilitis**
chylo- (pre) .... **cheilo-**
chyloplasty .... **cheiloplasty**
chyr- (pre) .... **chir-**
chyro- (pre) .... **chiro-**
chyropodist .... **chiropodist**
chyropractic .... **chiropractic**
ciatic nerve .... **sciatic nerve**
ciclazocen .... **cyclazocine**
ciclic AMP .... **cyclic AMP**
ciclopropane .... **cyclopropane**
cidderosis .... **siderosis**
cifilitic .... **syphilitic**
cigmoid flexure .... **sigmoid flexure**
cigmoydiscope .... **sigmoidoscope**
cignal node .... **signal node**
cignificant pathology ....
.... **significant pathology**
cignificence .... **significance**
ciklothimic .... **cyclothymic**
cilhouette .... **silhouette**
cillium .... **cilium****
cilyary body .... **ciliary body**
cimptomatology .... **symptomatology**
cimtum .... **symptom**
cimulate .... **simulate****
cincope .... **syncope**
cindrome .... **syndrome**
cinergism .... **synergism**

cingle hairlip .... **single harelip**
cinnovial .... **synovial**
cinosis .... **cyanosis**
Cintex .... **Syntex**
cinthesis .... **synthesis**
cinusitis .... **sinusitis**
cirebral cranials ...... **cerebral cranials**
ciringe .... **syringe**
cirvical erosion .... **cervical erosion**
cissed .... **cyst**
cisstitis .... **cystitis**
cist- (pre) .... **cyst-**
cistectomy .... **cystectomy**
cisti- (pre) .... **cysti-**
cistic duck .... **cystic duct**
cistic-fibrosis .... **cystic fibrosis**
cisto- (pre) .... **cysto-**
cistography .... **cystography**
cistole .... **systole**
cistoma .... **cystoma**
citakrome .... **cytochrome**
citameggalovirus ...... **cytomegalovirus**
cite- (pre) .... **cyt-**
citescope .... **cytoscope**
cito- (pre) .... **cyto-**
citoeskeleton .... **cytoskeleton**
citogenetics .... **cytogenetics**
citology .... **sitology****
citoplasm .... **cytoplasm**
citoxin .... **cytotoxin**
cittoglobulin .... **cytoglobulin**
claufoot .... **clawfoot**
clavvikul/o- (pre) .... **clavicul/o-**
clawdication .... **claudication**
clawstrofobia .... **claustrophobia**
claymant .... **claimant**
cleerance .... **clearance**
clinacal psychology ....
.... **clinical psychology**
cliniccal thermometer ....
.... **clinical thermometer**
clinnic .... **clinic**
clinnical dextran .... **clinical dextran**
clipp .... **clip**
clittoris .... **clitoris**
cloan .... **clone**
cloksicillin .... **cloxacillin**
cloniphene .... **clomiphene**

18

cloopeine .... **clupeine**
clor- (pre) .... **chlor-**
cloraform .... **chloroform**
clorakeen .... **chloroquine**
clorifill .... **chlorophyll**
clorimine-T .... **chloramine-T**
cloro- (pre) .... **chloro-**
clott .... **clot**
clozed circulatory system ....
.... **closed circulatory system**
clubing .... **clubbing**
clusster headache .... **cluster headache**
clyint-centered psychotherapy ....
..... **client-centered psychotherapy**
clymakteric .... **climacteric**
co-agyalated protein ....
.... **coagulated protein**
cobbalamin ....
.... **cobalamin** or **cobalamine**
cocanism .... **cocainism**
cocksix .... **coccyx**
coco .... **cocoa**
cocsa .... **coxa**
codd-liver oil .... **cod-liver oil**
codeen .... **codeine**
coebalt .... **cobalt**
coecane .... **cocaine**
coed call .... **code call**
co-enzime .... **coenzyme**
coetransport .... **cotransport**
co-faktor .... **cofactor**
cofee .... **coffee**
coff .... **cough**
coggnative psychology ....
.... **cognitive psychology**
Cohen biopsy .... **cone biopsy**
coinshurance .... **co-insurance**
cokaine .... **cocaine**
cokcidiodes immitis ....
.... *Coccidioides immitis*
coksyg/o- (pre) .... **coccyg/o-**
colajenolytic .... **collagenolytic**
colapse .... **collapse**
cole .... **cold**
Coles .... **Colles****
cole tar .... **coal tar**
colickee .... **colicky**
coligen .... **collagen**

colirium .... **collyrium**
collarectal cancer .... **colorectal cancer**
collds .... **colds****
colled therapy .... **cold therapy**
collegin diseases ..... **collagen diseases**
collera .... **cholera**
Collgate-Hoit .... **Colgate-Hoyt**
collic .... **colic**
collidgen vascular disease ....
.... **collagen vascular disease**
colliflower ear .... **cauliflower ear**
collim .... **column****
collinergic .... **cholinergic**
collitis .... **colitis**
collosinth .... **colocynth**
colls .... **coles****
colodion .... **collodion**
colone .... **colon**
colorbone .... **collarbone**
Cols .... **Colles****
colsore .... **cold sore**
colum .... **collum****
coluny .... **colony**
colytis .... **colitis**
comand neuron ..... **command neuron**
comdon .... **condom**
comeedo .... **comedo**
comepressed air sickness ....
.... **compressed air sickness**
comisura .... **commissura**
comma .... **coma**
commpact bone .... **compact bone**
commpensitory reaction ....
.... **compensatory reaction**
commplacation .... **complication**
commplex .... **complex**
commpreehensive medical
insurance ....
.... **comprehensive medical
insurance**
commpromised host ....
.... **compromised host**
comon cold .... **common cold**
compatable .... **compatible**
comyounity psychology ....
.... **community psychology**
comyunicable .... **communicable**
conaught .... **Connaught**

condile .... **condyle**
conective tissue ...... **connective tissue**
confeinment .... **confinement**
conjagal........................... **conjugal**
conjestion.......................... **congestion**
conkreetion .... **concretion**
conncha................................. **concha**
conndensation .... **condensation**
connducting portion ....
.... **conducting portion**
connfusion .... **confusion**
connjunctavitis.............. **conjunctivitis**
connservitive treatment ....
.... **conservative treatment**
connstitootional psychology...........
.... **constitutional psychology**
connstricter .... **constrictor**
connsulting sychology....................
.... **consulting psychology**
connsumtion .... **consumption**
conntact.............................. **contact****
conntact dermatitis ....
..........................**contact dermatitis**
conntaminent .... **contaminant**
conntract ....**contract****
conntraseptive .... **contraceptive**
conntrast .... **contrast**
conntrol.................................. **control**
conntusion........................... **contusion**
connvalessent................ **convalescent**
connvulshin.......................**convulsion**
conseive .... **conceive**
consentrate .... **concentrate**
consept .... **concept**
conshence .... **conscience****
conshus .... **conscious****
constapation .... **constipation**
contanent............................ **continent**
conteraction time .... **contraction time**
conter irritant .... **counterirritant**
contracoop .... **contrecoup**
contratransport .... **countertransport**
convursion disorder ....
......................**conversion disorder**
coomadin .... **Coumadin**
coper .... **copper**
coprafilia .... **coprophilia**

coranery artery......... **coronary artery**
corda .... **chorda**
cordination .... **coordination**
corective .... **corrective**
cored clamp .... **cord clamp**
coreeza................................. **coryza**
corelation .... **correlation**
corepusel ....**corpuscle**
coretex .... **cortex**
corinary artery bypass ....
................**coronary artery bypass**
cornary occlusion ....
.... **coronary occlusion**
corne .... **corn**
cornew .... **cornu**
cornia .... **cornea**
cornyal reflex .... **corneal reflex**
cornybacterium....... *Corynebacterium*
corola .... **corolla**
corpse callosum .... **corpus callosum**
corr..................................... **cor****
corrdotomy .... **cordotomy**
corronary........................ **coronary****
corroner............................ **coroner****
corr temperature .... **core temperature**
corrticoetropin .... **corticotropin**
cortacal .... **cortical**
cortakotropin releasing hormone ....
.... **corticotropin releasing
hormone**
corticko- (pre)........................**cortico-**
corunnary heart disease ....
.... **coronary heart disease**
coryidea ....**chorioidea**
cossed effectiveness ....
............................**cost effectiveness**
cossmid .... **cosmid**
cossto- (pre).............................. **costo-**
cote ....**coat**
coton .... **cotton**
cottin ball .... **cotton ball**
counsultation.................. **consultation**
counterceptive foam ....
.... **contraceptive foam**
countra- (pre)........................ **contra-**
countrindicated .... **contraindicated**
cowching............................. **couching**

Incorrect	Correct
cownter	counter
cowntercurrent multiplier system	countercurrent multiplier system
cowpocks	cowpox
coytal	coital
cozmetic surgery	cosmetic surgery
cpr	CPR
crabblouse	crab louse
cradel	cradle
crak	crack
crammp	cramp
crane- (pre)	crani-
craneal	cranial
craneal cavity	cranial cavity
cranectomy	craniectomy
craneo- (pre)	cranio-
craneograph	craniograph
craneopathy	craniopathy
crappyulent	crapulent
craynium	cranium
creeck	crick
creesol	cresol
creetinism	cretinism
creetin phosphate	creatine phosphate
crennation	crenation
creppatation	crepitation
cressed	crest
cressent	crescent
cretinine	creatinine**
cri- (pre)	cry-
cribb death	crib death
crikoid cartilage	cricoid cartilage
crio- (pre)	cryo-
criobirth	cryobirth
criocautery	cryocautery
criosergery	cryosurgery
cripling	crippling
cripptogenic	cryptogenic
cript- (pre)	crypt-
criptic	cryptic
cripto- (pre)	crypto-
criptoccocosis	cryptococcosis
crisotherapy	chrysotherapy
crissis	crisis

Incorrect	Correct
crissta	crista
crittacil	critical
cromasome	chromosome
cromat- (pre)	chromat-
cromatin	chromatin
cromato- (pre)	chromato-
cromeum	cromium
cronic	chronic
croock	crook
croop	croup
crosbridge	cross-bridge
cross-ekstensor reflex	cross-extensor reflex
cross-eyes	crossed eyes
croun	crown
croutch	crotch
cruch	crutch
crushal	crucial
cruss	crus**
crussed	crust**
crybank	cryobank
cuf	cuff
culchural alienation	cultural alienation
culchure	culture
cullaps therapy	collapse therapy
culldoscopy	culdoscopy
culloid	colloid
cullor blindness	color blindness
cullostomy bag	colostomy bag
culp- (pre)	colp-
culpitis	colpitis
culpo- (pre)	colpo-
culposcope	colposcope
culpyrinter	colpeurynter
culteral relativism	cultural relativism
cumbat fatigue	combat fatigue
cumpensation	compensation
cumplement	complement**
cumplete blood count	complete blood count
cumplex carbohydrate	complex carbohydrate
cumpliance	compliance
cumpliment	compliment**
cumposite	composite

Incorrect	Correct	Incorrect	Correct
cumpound fracture .... **compound fracture**		cushion's disease ... **Cushing's disease**	
cumpress .... **compress**		cusspid .... **cuspid**	
cumpulsion .... **compulsion**		cutecle .... **cuticle**	
cumputerized aksial tomography .... .. **computerized axial tomography**		cutt .... **cut**	
cumunity hospital .... **community hospital**		cyanno- (pre) .... **cyano-**	
cuncurant therapy .... **concurrent therapy**		cycklothyme .... **cyclothyme**	
cundiloma .... **condyloma**		cyderosis .... **siderosis**	
cundition .... **condition**		cyderotic nodules ... **siderotic nodules**	
cundrum .... **condom**		cyklic GMP .... **cyclic GMP**	
cunductive heering loss .... **conductive hearing loss**		cylent carsinoma ..... **silent carcinoma**	
cungectiva .... **conjectiva**		cymbiosis .... **symbiosis**	
cungenital .... **congenital**		cymmetrical .... **symmetrical**	
cuniform .... **cuneiform**		cymultaneous .... **simultaneous**	
cunilingus .... **cunnilingus**		cynchronous .... **synchronous**	
cunjoin therapy .... **conjoint therapy**		cyncope .... **syncope**	
cunnective tishue cells .... **connective tissue cells**		cyndrome .... **syndrome**	
cunsangwinity .... **consanguinity**		cynergism .... **synergism**	
cuntajious .... **contagious**		cynergy .... **synergy**	
cuntraction .... **contraction**		cynoauricular .... **sinoauricular**	
cuntrol system .... **control system**		Cyntex .... **Syntex**	
cunvergence .... **convergence**		cynthesis .... **synthesis**	
cureall .... **cure-all**		cynusoidal .... **sinusoidal**	
curent .... **current**		-cysst (suff) .... **-cyst**	
curinary care unit .... **coronary care unit**		cysteen .... **cystine**	
curitive .... **curative**		cystem .... **system**	
currare .... **curare**		cystole .... **systole**	
currebrospinal fluid .... **cerebrospinal fluid**		cystomatic .... **systematic**	
currett .... **curette**		cytollogy .... **cytology****	
currona .... **corona**		cytrate of magnesia .... **citrate of magnesia**	
		cytte .... **cite****	
		cyuboid .... **cuboid**	
		cyumulative drugs .... **cumulative drugs**	
		cyure .... **cure**	
		cyutaneous .... **cutaneous**	

D

Incorrect	Correct	Incorrect	Correct
dactil .... **dactyl**		Dallkon sheeld .... **Dalkon shield**	
dactil- (pre) .... **dactyl-**		daltinism .... **daltonism**	
dactilo- (pre) .... **dactylo- (pre)**		danndruf .... **dandruff**	
dactilology .... **dactylology**		darc adaptation .... **dark adaptation**	
dait sugar .... **date sugar**		darvan .... **Darvon**	
dakry/o- (pre) .... **dacry/o-**		datta .... **data**	

Incorrect	Correct
dc	DC
dds	DDS
ddsc	DDSc
debbility	debility
decensitization	desensitization
ded space	dead space
dee- (pre)	de-
Dee and C	D & C
deebridement	debridement
deecompression	decompression
deefect	defect
deefens mechanism	defense mechanism
deefermation	deformation
deeglutition	deglutition
deehidrocorticosterone	dehydrocorticosterone
deekrepit	decrepit
deelimit	delimit
deemonology	demonology
deeoxyheemoglobin	deoxyhemoglobin
deepressive sychosis	depressive psychosis
deesent	descent**
deesoksyephedrine	desoxyephedrine
deetached retina	detached retina
deeviance	deviance
deffecation	defecation
deffibrilator	defibrillator
defficit	deficit**
deffness	deafness
deff psychology	depth psychology
deffusion equilibrium	diffusion equilibrium
def muteness	deaf muteness
degestive system	digestive system
degstran	dextran**
degstrose	dextrose**
dehidration	dehydration
dehyssence	dehiscence
dejeneration	degeneration
dejenerative	degenerative
dekongestant	decongestant
deksamethasone	dexamethasone
dekubitus ulcer	decubitus ulcer
dekyubation	decubation

Incorrect	Correct
delation and evacuation	dilation and evacuation
dellerium tremens	delirium tremens
delltoid	deltoid
deloosional syndrome	delusional syndrome
demmentia precox	dementia praecox
Demmerol	Demerol
demmulcent	demulcent
denchures	dentures
deng	dengue**
denyal	denial
denndrite	dendrite
dennt- (pre)	dent-
denntal extraction forceps	dental extraction forceps
denntical	denticle
denntist	dentist
dennto- (pre)	dento-
denntofashal	dentofacial
dentall technician	dental technician
denteen	dentin or dentine
dentees	dentes**
dentefriss	dentifrice
dentel flos	dental floss
dentestry	dentistry
dentil drill	dental drill
dentill	dental
dentl surgery	dental surgery
denttal higienist	dental hygienist
denty- (pre)	denti-
dentyfriss	dentifrice
deoksyribonucleic acid	deoxyribonucleic acid
dependancy	dependency
depiggmenting agent	depigmenting agent
depilittory	depilatory
depollorization	depolarization
depot-provera	Depo-Provera
deppendence	dependence
deppression	depression
depresive nurosis	depressive neurosis
dept psychology	depth psychology
depursonilization	depersonalization

dermattofytosis .... **dermatophytosis**
dermetology .... **dermatology**
dermil sheath .... **dermal sheath**
-dermiss (suff) .... **-dermis**
dermititis .... **dermatitis****
dermmatotherapy ..... **dermatotherapy**
dermoyd cist .... **dermoid cyst**
-derrm (suff) .... **-derm**
derrmato- (pre) .... **dermato-**
desiduma .... **deciduoma****
Dess daughter .... **Des daughter**
dessending colon ... **descending colon**
dessmosome .... **desmosome**
dessoxicorticosterone ....
.... **desoxycorticosterone**
dessucate .... **desiccate****
desypramine .... **desipramine**
det ....**DET**
deth certificate .... **death certificate**
detirioration .... **deterioration**
detoksification .... **detoxification**
detreetis............................... **detritus**
dettumessence .... **detumescence**
deveated septum ...... **deviated septum**
devellopmental psychology ....
.... **developmental psychology**
devyation .... **deviation**
dexadrine .... **Dexedrine**
Deximyl .... **Dexamyl**
dextramphetamine sulfate ....
...... **dextroamphetamine sulfate**
dextrenagenic enzyme ....
.... **dextrinogenic enzyme**
dexxtrin .... **dextrin****
dexxtro- (pre) .... **dextro-**
deziner drug .... **designer drug**
dezm/o- (pre) .... **desm/o-**
diafisis .... **diaphysis**
diafram .... **diaphragm****
diallysis machine .... **dialysis machine**
diaminase .... **deaminase**
diaretic .... **diuretic**
diatician .... **dietician**
dibbucain .... **dibucaine**
dibinese .... **Diabinese**
dibridement .... **debridement**
Dickreed .... **Dick-Read**

dicompression sickness ....
.... **decompression sickness**
didotyrosine .... **diiodotyrosine**
diebeetes insipidus ....
.... **diabetes insipidus**
diegnossis-related group ....
.... **diagnosis-related group**
diel ....**Dial**
dierhea .... **diarrhea****
dietheesis .... **diathesis**
diethilstylbestrole ... **diethylstilbestrol**
difanoscope .... **diaphanoscope**
difense.................................. **defense**
difenylhydantoin ...... **diphenyldantoin**
diferentally abeld.... **differently abled**
difformity .... **deformity**
dificiency disease ....
.... **deficiency disease**
difrential diagnosis ....
.... **differential diagnosis**
diftheria....................... **diphtheria****
difusion .... **diffusion**
diggitalin .... **digitalin****
digittal nerve .... **digital nerve**
dijestion .... **digestion**
dijetalis .... **digitalis****
dijit..**digit**
dikoomarin .... **dicoumarin**
dilirium .... **delirium**
dillantin................................. **Dilantin**
dillation and currettage ....
.... **dilation and curettage**
dillute .... **dilute****
dilusion .... **delusion****
dimentia .... **dementia**
dimmentians .... **dementians**
diothermy .... **diathermy**
dipendent pursonality ....
.... **dependent personality**
diper rash .... **diaper rash**
diplacocus .... **diplococcus**
dipplococci .... **diplococci**
dipploid................................. **diploid****
dipplomate .... **diplomate**
dipplopia .... **diplopia****
dippressive reaction ....
.... **depressive reaction**

dipps/o- (pre) .... **dips/o-**
dipressant .... **depressant**
dis- (pre) .... **dys-**
disasociative disorder ....
.... **dissociative disorder**
disect .... **dissect**
disepam .... **diazepam**
disfunction .... **dysfunction**
disilution .... **dissolution****
disinnhibition .... **disinhibition**
diskreet .... **discrete****
diskus .... **discus****
disleksia .... **dyslexia**
dismennorea .... **dysmenorrhea**
disociation reaction ....
.... **dissociation reaction**
disorrientation .... **disorientation**
disparenia .... **dyspareunia**
displasement .... **displacement**
dispnia .... **dyspnea**
diss- (pre) .... **dys-**
dissability .... **disability**
dissastole .... **diastole**
disscharge .... **discharge**
dissclose .... **disclose**
disscus .... **discuss****
dissentery .... **dysentery**
dissinfectant .... **disinfectant****
dissintegrate .... **disintegrate**
disslokation .... **dislocation**
dissorder .... **disorder**
disspensery .... **dispensary**
dissplaced aggression ....
.... **displaced aggression**
disst/o- (pre) .... **dist/o-**
disstal .... **distal****
disstemper .... **distemper**
distil .... **distill****
distrafy .... **dystrophy**
dithermy machine ....
.... **diathermy machine**
dithiltryptamine .... **diethyltryptamine**
ditotherapy .... **dietotherapy**
divertikulossis .... **diverticulosis****
divverticular disease ....
.... **diverticular disease**
dizease .... **disease****

dizolve .... **dissolve**
dizzygotic twins .... **dizygotic twins**
dizzyness .... **dizziness**
dobble vision .... **double vision**
Docter of Medicine ....
.... **Doctor of Medicine**
doenee .... **donee****
doktor .... **doctor**
dollor .... **dolor****
domanint hemisphere ....
.... **dominant hemisphere**
domminant geen .... **dominant gene**
doner insemmination ....
.... **donor insemination**
donnor .... **donor****
doodenum .... **duodenum**
doorsal .... **dorsal**
dooshing .... **douching**
dopimine .... **dopamine**
dores/o- (pre) .... **dors/o-**
dorsil dispepsia .... **dorsal dyspepsia**
dosse .... **dose****
dossimetry .... **dosimetry**
doss-response fenomenon ....
.... **dose-response phenomenon**
dowegers hump ...... **dowager's hump**
Down's syndrome .... **Down syndrome**
doxyribose .... **deoxyribose**
dr .... **Dr.**
drakontisis .... **dracontiasis**
dramimine .... **Dramamine**
drane .... **drain**
drayn toob .... **drain tube**
dreem .... **dream**
dresing .... **dressing**
DRGr .... **DRG**
droopsy .... **dropsy****
dropplet infection ... **droplet infection**
drugg .... **drug**
drugist .... **druggist**
dubble helix .... **double helix**
ducktis deferens .... **ductus deferens**
ducless gland .... **ductless gland**
dudden/o- (pre) .... **duoden/o-**
dudenal ulcer .... **duodenal ulcer**
dukt .... **duct**
duktus .... **ductus**

Incorrect	Correct	Incorrect	Correct
dule innervation	**duel innervation**	dyalisis	**dialysis**
dummping	**dumping**	dyathurmy knife	**diathermy knife**
dumping sindrome	**dumping syndrome**	dybensoxazepines	**dibenzoxazepines**
Dupont	**Du Pont**	dydyoxyinosine	**dideoxyinosine**
durm- (pre)	**derm-**	dyestolic pressure	**diastolic pressure**
durma- (pre)	**derma-**	dyet	**diet****
-durma (suff)	**-derma**	dyhidrostreptomycin	**dihydrostreptomycin**
durmabrasion	**dermabrasion**	dyibetes	**diabetes**
durmal	**dermal**	dyiforesis	**diaphoresis**
durmata- (pre)	**dermata-**	dymmethiltryptamine	**dimethyltryptamine**
-durmata (suff)	**-dermata**	dyper rash	**diaper rash**
durmatitis	**dermatitis****	dyplegia	**diplegia**
durmatology	**dermatology**	dyshuria	**dysuria**
durmatosis	**dermatosis****	dyspajia	**dysphagia****
durmetone	**dermatome**	dyspeppsia	**dyspepsia**
-durmis (suff)	**-dermis**	dysslalia	**dyslalia**
-durmm (suff)	**-derm**	dysulferam	**disulfuram**
durmo- (pre)	**dermo-**	dy therapy	**dye therapy**
durra matter	**dura mater**	dyvergence	**divergence**
dwafism	**dwarfism**	dyvurticulitis	**diverticulitis****
dyabetes melitus	**diabetes mellitus**		
dyagnosis	**diagnosis****		

E

Incorrect	Correct	Incorrect	Correct
ealectrode	**electrode**	edeema	**edema**
earake	**earache**	edipal	**oedipal**
ear-drumm	**eardrum**	Edipus complex	**Oedipus complex**
ear-lobe	**earlobe**	eebrius	**ebrious****
eccdopic pregnancy	**ectopic pregnancy**	eeclampsia	**eclampsia**
ecclectic psychology	**eclectic psychology**	eeg arowsal	**EEG arousal**
ecco	**echo**	eejaculate	**ejaculate**
-ecctasis (suff)	**-ectasis**	-eel (suff)	**-eal**
eckography	**echography****	eelasstic	**elastic**
ecks-ray	**x-ray**	eelastic bandage	**elastic bandage**
ecksray mashine	**x-ray machine**	eelectric	**electric**
-ecktomy (suff)	**-ectomy**	eelectrical stimulation of the brain	**electrical stimulation of the brain**
ecktopic focus	**ectopic focus**	eelectrolite	**electrolyte**
ecreen gland	**eccrine gland**	eemedic	**emetic**
ecrine	**eccrine**	-eemia (suff)	**-emia**
ectaderm	**ectoderm****	eemulsification	**emulsification**
-eddema (suff)	**-edema**	eer	**ear**
eddestin	**edestin**		

Incorrect	Correct	Incorrect	Correct
eerect	**erect****	ekt- (pre)	ect-
eerwax	**ear wax**	-ektasia (suff)	-ectasia
eesential	**essential**	ekto- (pre)	ecto-
eesinophil	**eosinophil**	ektocornea	**ectocornea**
eesoffag/o- (pre)	**esophag/o-**	ektomorph	**ectomorph****
eesophigus	**esophagus**	ekwil	**equal**
eessential nootrients		ekwilibrium potential	
	essential nutrients		**equilibrium potential**
eether	**ether****	ekymosis	**ecchymosis**
eetholigy	**ethology****	elafantisis	**elephantiasis**
eeu- (pre)	**eu-**	elasstin	**elastin**
eevacuator	**evacuator**	elboe	**elbow**
efacement	**effacement**	el-dopa	**L-dopa**
efect	**effect****	elecktrocaudery	**electrocautery**
efedrine	**ephedrine**	elecktron	**electron**
efektor	**effector**	elecktrotherepy	**electrotherapy**
effective disorder		electergraph	**electrograph**
	affective disorder	electrencefalograph	
eflerescence	**efflorescence**		**electroencephalograph**
efrent nuron	**efferent neuron**	ELEESA	**ELISA**
egaculate	**ejaculate**	elektrocardiogram	
eggoism	**egoism****		**electrocardiogram****
eggotism	**egotism****	elektrolysis	**electrolysis**
eggsplosion	**explosion**	elektroserjery	**electrosurgery**
egoe	**ego**	elevil	**Elavil**
egsamination	**examination**	elifantman's disease	
egsanthematous	**exanthematous**		**elephantman's disease**
egsogenous	**exogenous****	eligsir	**elixir**
egstension	**extension**	elimentary	**elementary****
egzema	**eczema**	ell-doper	**L-dopa**
ekg	**EKG**	ellectr- (pre)	**electr-**
ekocardiography		ellectra complex	**Electra complex**
	echocardiography**	ellectro- (pre)	**electro-**
eksamine	**examine**	ellectrocardiophonogram	
eksedontist	**exodontist**		**electrocardiophonogram**
eksistential sychotherapy		Ellkins' Sin	**Elkins-Sinn**
	existential psychotherapy	elsd	**LSD**
eksitation	**excitation**	Ely Lilly	**Eli Lilly**
ekskretion	**excretion**	emashiation	**emaciation**
ekspecctant	**expectant**	emassculation	**emasculation**
ekspectorant	**expectorant**	embreology	**embryology**
ekspload	**explode**	embrioe	**embryo**
ekspressivity	**expressivity**	embulus	**embolus**
ekstenders	**extenders**	-emeesis (suff)	**-emesis**
ekstenser	**extensor**	emenation	**emanation**
eksternal	**external**	emerjency room	**emergency room**
ekstrinsic cloting pathway		emm- (pre)	**em-**
	extrinsic clotting pathway	emmbolism	**embolism**

Incorrect	Correct	Incorrect	Correct

emmergency medical service ....

.... **emergency medical service**

emminentia .... **eminentia**

emmolient .... **emollient**

emmpiric risk .... **empiric risk**

emmunomodulators ....

.... **immunomodulators**

emoshion...................... **emotion**

emoshonal instability reaction ....

...... **emotional instability reaction**

emprin .... **Empirin**

emurjency medical technician.........

..... **emergency medical technician**

enammel .... **enamel**

enavate .... **enervate****

encefal/o- (pre) .... **encephal/o-**

encoherence .... **incoherence**

endacrinatherepy ... **endocrinotherapy**

endakarditis .... **endocarditis**

endaplazmic reticulum ....

.... **endoplasmic reticulum**

endascope .... **endoscope**

enddosytosis .... **endocytosis**

endecrine gland .... **endocrine gland**

endedentist .... **endodontist****

endeema .... **endema****

endemorf .... **endomorph****

endetrakeal tube ... **endotracheal tube**

endicreen system ... **endocrine system**

endidurm .... **endoderm****

endimeetriosis .... **endometriosis**

endokrinology .... **endocrinology**

endorfin............................ **endorphin**

endpeptedase .... **endopeptidase**

endremeetreal carcinoma.................

.... **endometrial carcinoma**

enduration .... **induration**

eneureesis .... **enuresis**

enfirmity .... **infirmity**

enfysema .... **emphysema**

engina pectoris .... **angina pectoris**

enhanncer........................... **enhancer**

enjineering psychology ....

.... **engineering psychology**

enn- (pre) .... **en-**

-enncefalia (suff) .... **-encephalia**

enncrust............................. **encrust****

ennd/o- (pre) .... **end/o-**

enndemick......................... **endemic****

enndodonticks .... **endodontics****

ennema................................ **enema****

ennervation .... **enervation**

ennhansement .... **enhancement**

ennt/o- (pre)............................. **ent/o-**

ennter/o- (pre)...................... **enter/o-**

ennterostomy .... **enterostomy**

ennzyme induction ....

.... **enzyme induction**

enpyeema .... **empyema**

ensephalitis .... **encephalitis**

ensimology .... **enzymology**

entaviral diseases.........................

.... **enteroviral diseases**

entederm .... **entoderm****

Entemeeba histolitica ....

.... ***Entamoeba histolytica***

entercostal muscle ....

.... **intercostal muscle**

enterstitial fluid .... **interstitial fluid**

entertrigo........................... **intertrigo**

entestinal juice .... **intestinal juice**

entirior .... **anterior**

entrakinese .... **enterokinese**

entrascleral .... **intrascleral**

entravenous therapy ....

.... **intravenous therapy**

entrinsic factor .... **intrinsic factor**

entritis .... **enteritis**

entroseal .... **enterocele**

entubation .... **intubation**

enyuresis .... **enuresis**

enzime.................................. **enzyme**

enzymm-linked immunosorbent

assay ....

... **enzyme-linked immunosorbent**
assay

epedemic .... **epidemic****

epedermofytosis ..... **epidermophytosis**

epefysis .... **epiphysis**

epekanthic fold .... **epicanthic fold**

epestaxis .... **epistaxis**

epethilioma .... **epithelioma**

ephithelial cells.......... **epithelial cells**

epickanthus .... **epicanthus**

epiddermophyton ..... **epidermophyton**

epididdimis .... **epididymis**

epidimeology .... epidemiology
epiglotis .... epiglottis
epijastrium .... epigastrium
episeotimy .... episiotomy
epissode .... episode
epistaksis .... epistaxis
epitheelium .... epithelium
eplepsy .... epilepsy
epp- or eppi- (pre) .... ep- or epi-
eppidemic .... epidemic**
eppidermis .... epidermis
eppilepsey .... epilepsy
eppinefrine .... epinephrine
eppisi/o- (pre) ....episi/o-
Eppsom salts .... Epsom salts
Epsteen-Bar syndrome ....
.... Epstein-Barr syndrome
equil .... equal
equinal .... Equanil
erbal remedies .... herbal remedies
ere canal .... ear canal
erectation .... eructation**
ereethro- (pre) ....erythro-
ereethromycin .... erythromycin
ereethrosyte sedimentation rate ....
.... erythrocyte sedimentation rate
erektile dysfunction ....
.... erectile dysfunction
ergatherapy .... ergotherapy
ergensy .... urgency
ergo .... ergot
erisipelas .... erysipelas
eritheema ....erythema**
erithropoesis .... erythropoiesis
-erjic (suff)........................ -ergic
Erlick .... Ehrlich
errector........................... erector
errotic............................. erotic**
erroto- (pre) ....eroto-
erruct................................ eruct**
errythrocyte.................... erythrocyte
erthropotin .... erythropoietin
erythrows ....erythrose
esential amino acids ....
.... essential amino acids
esherishia ....escherichia
esofajeal orifice .... esophageal orifice
esscape ....escape

essthezi/o- (pre) .... esthesi/o-
esstriol................................ estriol
esstrone .... estrone
esstrus .... estrus**
esteradiole .... estradiol
estergen .... estrogen
estherin .... estrin
estrase .... esterase
estrus .... estrous**
ethel chloride .... ethyl chloride
ethil .... ethyl
ethilene oxide .... ethylene oxide
ethleen ....ethylene
ethmoyd .... ethmoid
etyo- (pre) .... etio-
etyology .... etiology
euforia .... euphoria**
eurine .... urine
eurology .... urology
evakuation .... evacuation
evvaluation .... evaluation
ewe- (pre) .... oo-
exacise .... exercise**
exalation .... exhalation
excapism .... escapism
ex-chromasomal aberration ....
.... x-chromosomal aberration
ex chromosome .... x-chromosome
execrin gland .... exocrine gland
exestential nurosis ....
.... existential neurosis
exibitionism .... exhibitionism
exitatory synapse ....
.... excitatory synapse
exite .... excite
exkriment .... excrement
exlinkage........................... x-linkage
exoddontics .... exodontics
exothalmic goiter ....
.... exophthalmic goiter
exparatory reserve volume ....
.... expiratory reserve volume
expenders .... expanders
experamint .... experiment
experation .... expiration
experremental psychology ....
.... experimental psychology
exray machine .... x-ray machine

Incorrect	Correct	Incorrect	Correct

ex-ray technician ..... **x-ray technician**
exsedrin.............................. **Excedrin**
exsision .... **excision**
exsitibility .... **excitability**
extercellular fluid ....
.... **extracellular fluid**
extireor................................ **exterior**
extraktion .... **extraction**
extravert .... **extrovert**
extrehapetic .... **extrahepatic**
extremmity .... **extremity**
exturnal cuniform ....
.... **external cuneiform**
exx/o- (pre) ....**ex/o-**
exxaminning room .. **examining room**
exxchange transfusion ....
.... **exchange transfusion**
exxercise .... **exercise****
exxoginous .... **exogenous****
exxon .... **exon****
exxosytosis .... **exocytosis**
exxpectent .... **expectant**
exxpert .... **expert**
exxplode .... **explode**
exxploritory surgery ....

.... **exploratory surgery**
exxpulsion........................ **expulsion**
exxternal .... **external**
exxtra- (pre).............................**extra-**
exxtrakt .... **extract**
exxtreemitas .... **extremitas**
ey .... **eye**
eyball .... **eyeball**
-eydan (suff) ....**-idan**
-eyea (suff) .... **-ia**
Eye and D .... **I and D**
eye lash .... **eyelash**
eyelets of Langerhans ....
.... **islets of Langerhans**
eyeris.. **iris**
eyeritis .... **iritis**
-eyetis (suff) .... **-itis**
eylid .... **eyelid**
eyodotherapy .... **iodotherapy**
eyris .... **iris**
eysocket .... **eye socket**
eysolation ward .... **isolation ward**
-eytis (suff) .... **-itis**
eytuck .... **eye tuck**
-eyv (suff) ....**-ive**

F

fac- (pre) .... **phac-**
facees .... **facies****
facillitation .... **facilitation**
fack- (pre) .... **phak-**
facko- (pre) .... **phako-**
fackulty .... **faculty**
faclift...................................... **facelift**
faco- (pre) .... **phaco-**
facter ....**factor**
fage .... **phage**
fagg- (pre) .... **phag-**
-fagia (suff) .... **-phagia**
-fagic (suff) .... **-phagic**
fago- (pre) .... **phago-**
-fagy (suff) .... **-phagy**
fakter eight or fakter VIII ....
.... **factor eight** or **factor VIII**
faktitious disorders ....
.... **factitious disorders**
falango- (pre) .... **phalango-**
falanx .... **phalanx**
falce labor ....**false labor**
fall/o- (pre) .... **phallo-**
fallic simbol .... **phallic symbol**
falls teeth .... **false teeth**
falopian tube .... **fallopian tube**
falss pregnancy .... **false pregnancy**
falure .... **failure**
famaly practioner.........................
.... **family practitioner**
famely .... **family**
famly doctor .... **family doctor**
fammily medicine .... **family medicine**
fantisy .... **fantasy**

Incorrect	Correct
fantom limb	**phantom limb**
farinjo- (pre)	**pharyngo-**
farinx	**pharynx**
farmaceutical	**pharmaceutical**
farmacist	**pharmacist**
farmacologist	**pharmacologist**
farmacology	**pharmacology**
farmacopoeia	**pharmacopoeia**
farmacy	**pharmacy**
farrenhite	**Fahrenheit**
farring- (pre)	**pharyng-**
farsitedness	**farsightedness**
faryngeal	**pharyngeal****
faryngitis	**pharyngitis**
fase	**phase**
fashe	**phage**
fashial nerve	**facial nerve**
-fasia (suff)	**-phasia**
fasia lata	**fascia lata**
faskial	**fascial****
fassia	**fascia****
fassilitated diffusion	
	facilitated diffusion
fassility	**facility**
fasskiculi	**fasciculi**
fasstidious	**fastidious**
fastijium	**fastigium**
fateegue	**fatigue**
fatee liver	**fatty liver**
fathe healer	**faith healer**
fatil	**fatal****
fatt	**fat**
faty acids	**fatty acids**
fawlse rib	**false rib**
fayse	**face**
faylure	**failure**
faynt	**faint****
fayvus	**favus**
fazic	**phasic**
feable	**feeble****
feadback	**feedback**
feaver therapy	**fever therapy**
febrefuge	**febrifuge**
feckund	**fecund**
feebri- (pre)	**febri-**
feebrile	**febrile****
feemale	**female**
feemur	**femur**

Incorrect	Correct
feer	**fear**
feeral	**feral****
feeses	**feces****
feet/o- (pre)	**fet/o-**
feetal alcohol syndrome	
	fetal alcohol syndrome
feetus	**fetus**
feever	**fever**
feinting	**fainting**
fekal sofeners	**fecal softeners**
felashio	**fellatio**
felbogram	**phlebogram**
femmer/o- (pre)	**femor/o-**
femminine	**feminine**
femminin hygiene	
	feminine hygiene
femmoral nerve	**femoral nerve**
fenacetin	**phenacetin**
fenel	**fennel****
fenistration	**fenestration**
fennel salicylate	**phenyl salicylate**
fennol	**phenol**
fenocopy	**phenocopy**
fenoglycodal	**phenoglycodal**
fenomenon	**phenomenon**
fenothiazine	**phenothiazine**
fenyl	**phenyl****
fenylketonuria	**phenylketonuria**
feretin	**ferritin**
ferous	**ferrous**
ferrtility drug	**fertility drug**
ferst-degree burn	**first-degree burn**
fesster	**fester**
fetel distress	**fetal distress**
fettish	**fetish**
fettishism	**fetishism**
fevver blister	**fever blister**
fibbrinogen	**fibrinogen**
fibbroma	**fibroma**
fibbula	**fibula**
fiberepithelial tumor	
	fibroepithelial tumor
fibernolytic	**fibrinolytic**
fiberocistic breast	
	fibrocystic breast
fiberosarcoma	**fibrosarcoma**
fiberous	**fibrous****
fibraddenoma	**fibroadenoma**

Incorrect	Correct
fibralation	**fibrillation**
fibrasystic disease	
	fibrocystic disease
fibre	**fiber**
fibrocis	**fibrosis**
fibroes	**fibrose****
fibyul/o- (pre)	**fibul/o-**
figger-of-eight	**figure-of-eight**
-file (suff)	**-phile**
fileum	**filum****
-filiac (suff)	**-philiac**
fillament	**filament**
fillarysis	**filariasis**
filleng	**filling****
filltration	**filtration**
filtrum	**philtrum**
fingerr	**finger**
finnger bones	**finger bones**
firtilize	**fertilize**
fiscal medicine	**physical medicine**
fishon	**fission**
fishure	**fissure****
fisi- (pre)	**physi-**
fisic	**physic****
fisician liability	**physician liability**
fisio- (pre)	**physio-**
fisiological	**physiological**
fisiotherapy	**physiotherapy**
fisst	**fist**
fistyula	**fistula**
fisura	**fissura****
fite- (pre)	**phyt-**
fite-or-flight response	
	fight-or-flight response
fito- (pre)	**phyto-**
fitt	**fit**
fixd-fee	**fixed-fee**
fixxation	**fixation**
Fizer	**Pfizer**
fiziatricks	**physiatrics****
flachburn	**flashburn**
flagil	**Flagyl**
flajella	**flagella**
flamable	**flammable**
flapp	**flap**

Incorrect	Correct
flatened effect	**flattened effect**
flatt	**flat**
flattulence	**flatulence**
flattus	**flatus**
fleb/o- (pre)	**phleb/o-**
flebitis	**phlebitis**
flech	**flesh**
flecser muscle	**flexor muscle**
fleggmatic	**phlegmatic**
flegmonous	**phlegmonous**
fleks	**flex**
fleksyon	**flexion**
flem	**phlegm****
flemm	**phloem****
flexxer	**flexor****
flexxon reflex	**flexion reflex**
flikker	**flicker**
flite of ideas	**flight of ideas**
floe	**flow**
floch	**flush**
flooid	**fluid**
flooroscope	**fluoroscope**
floroscopy	**fluoroscopy**
floter	**floater**
floting rib	**floating rib**
flourine	**fluorine****
flucks	**flux****
flue	**flu****
fluktuate	**fluctuate**
fluxx	**flux****
flyte reaction	**flight reaction**
-fobe (suff)	**-phobe**
fobia	**phobia**
fobic	**phobic**
focis	**focus**
foebic reaction	**phobic reaction**
foke medicine	**folk medicine**
folickle	**follicle**
follecel-stimulating hormone	
	follicle-stimulating hormone
follic acid	**folic acid**
follin	**Folin**
folow-up	**follow-up**
foly catheter	**Foley catheter**
fome	**foam**

Incorrect	Correct
fonation	**phonation****
fonetic	**phonetic**
food poysoning	**food poisoning**
forarm	**forearm**
forchette	**fourchette**
foreceps	**forceps**
foremaldehyde	**formaldehyde**
foremative	**formative**
forign	**foreign**
formen	**foramen**
formilin	**formalin**
forr- (pre)	**fore-****
forrensic medicine	**forensic medicine**
forrhead	**forehead**
forseps	**forceps**
fosa	**fossa**
fosfeen	**phosphene****
fosforylase	**phosphorylase**
fosphate	**phosphate**
fosphoglucomutase	**phosphoglucomutase**
fotic	**photic**
foto- (pre)	**photo-**
fotogen	**photogen****
fotopic vision	**photopic vision**
fotopigment	**photopigment**
fotoreceptor	**photoreceptor**
foull	**foul**
fournix	**fornix**
fourplay	**foreplay**
four-profit	**for-profit**
fovee centralis	**fovea centralis**
fractcher reduction	**fracture reduction**
fraddicin	**fradicin**
frajile	**fragile**
frakture	**fracture**
frammbesia	**frambesia**
frea radical	**free radical**
freese	**freeze****
fren- (pre)	**phren-**
frenic	**phrenic**
freno- (pre)	**phreno-**
fridgid	**frigid**

Incorrect	Correct
fridgotherapy	**frigotherapy**
frijidity	**frigidity**
frikshun	**friction**
Froid	**Freud**
Froidian psychoanalysis	**freudian psychoanalysis**
frontel	**frontal**
frooctose	**fructose**
froot sugar	**fruit sugar**
frosen shoulder	**frozen shoulder**
frossbite	**frostbite**
frozzen section	**frozen section**
Frued	**Freud**
frunculus	**furunculus**
fruntal lobe	**frontal lobe**
frusstrated	**frustrated**
fryable mass	**friable mass**
ftalysulfathiazole	**phthalysulfalthiazole**
fuge	**fugue****
-fuje (suff)	**-fuge**
fulblown AIDS	**full-blown AIDS**
fungis	**fungus**
fungtionalism	**functionalism**
funjal infections	**fungal infections**
funjicides	**fungicides**
funktional disorder	**functional disorder**
funndus	**fundus**
funniculus	**funiculus**
furmention	**fermentation**
furning	**ferning**
furruncle	**furuncle**
furst aid	**first aid**
furtile days	**fertile days**
fybray	**fibrae**
fybrin	**fibrin**
fybro- (pre)	**fibro-**
fybroids	**fibroids**
fyla	**fila****
fylum terminate	**filum terminate**
fysically	**physically**
fysical therapy	**physical therapy**
fysiopathology	**physiopathology**
fyusion	**fusion**

G

Incorrect	Correct
gabba	**GABA**
gach	**gash**
gaite	**gait**
gaitkeeper	**gatekeeper**
galactoefagus	**galactophagous****
galaktosemia	**galactosemia**
galbladder	**gallbladder**
gallact/o- (pre)	**galact/o-**
gallactose	**galactose****
gama globbulin	**gamma globulin**
gamamminobutyric acid	**gamma-aminobutyric acid**
gameet	**gamete**
gammete intra-fallopian transfer	**gamete intra-fallopian transfer**
ganga	**ganja**
ganglean	**ganglion**
ganglya	**ganglia**
gangreen	**gangrene**
Ganntrism	**Gantrism**
Ganzer syndrome	**Ganser's syndrome**
gapp junction	**gap junction**
gargel	**gargle**
gashous	**gaseous**
gass	**gas**
gassdric ulcer	**gastric ulcer**
gasstr/o- (pre)	**gastr/o-**
gasstrectomy	**gastrectomy**
gasteric lavage	**gastric lavage**
gasterin	**gastrin**
gasterintestinal tract	**gastrointestinal tract**
gastrascope	**gastroscope**
gastrenteritis	**gastroenteritis**
gastrick juice	**gastric juice**
gastrittis	**gastritis**
gastrocknemus	**gastrocnemius**
gastrontorology	**gastroenterology**
gawl	**gall**
gawlstone	**gallstone**
gawze	**gauze****
gayze	**gaze****
gean therapy	**gene therapy**
Gee I series	**GI series**
geen	**gene**
geenetic counseling	**genetic counseling**
-geenic (suff)	**-genic**
geenomic DNA	**genomic DNA**
gelactotherapy	**galactotherapy**
gellatinous	**gelatinous**
genatype	**genotype**
genchian violet	**gentian violet**
Genentek	**Genentech**
gennder	**gender**
Genneral Practioner	**general practitioner**
genneric	**generic**
gennerral	**general**
-gennesis (suff)	**-genesis**
-gennetic (suff)	**-genetic**
gennettic	**genetic**
gennit/o- (pre)	**genit/o-**
genral anesthetic	**general anesthetic**
gental herpes	**genital herpes**
gentle warts	**genital warts**
gerr/o- (pre)	**ger/o-**
gerranial	**geranial****
germicidal lamp	**germicidal lamp**
gerrney	**gurney**
gerront/o- (pre)	**geront/o-**
gerrontology	**gerontology**
geshtalt	**gestalt**
gesstosis	**gestosis**
gfr	**GFR**
gibouss	**gibbus****
gibuss	**gibbous****
Gieger	**Geiger**
Giegy	**Geigy**
gifft	**GIFT**
gillt	**guilt**
ginecologist	**gynecologist**
ginek/o- (pre)	**gynec/o-**
ginetic engineering	**genetic engineering**
ginjiva	**gingiva**
giris	**gyrus****

gladdiolus .... **gladiolus**
glanddalar therapy ....
.... **glandular therapy**
glandeler .... **glandular****
glanduller system ....
.... **glandular system**
glandyala .... **glandula****
glandyular fever .... **glandular fever**
glanned .... **gland**
glanns .... **glands****
glewcocorticoid .... **glucocorticoid**
glukonogenesis .... **gluconeogenesis**
glic/o- (pre) .... **glyc/o-**
glicerin .... **glycerin**
glicoss/o- (pre) .... **glycos/o-**
glideing joint .... **gliding joint**
glidin .... **gliadin**
gliecolisis .... **glycolysis**
glikogenolysis .... **glycogenolysis**
gliserole .... **glycerol**
glisserogel .... **glycerogel**
globbin .... **globin****
globyulin .... **globulin**
glommeruler filtration rate ....
.... **glomerular filtration rate**
glomrule/o- (pre) .... **glomerul/o-**
glomuruloe nephritis ....
.... **glomerulonephritis**
gloocose .... **glucose****
glootaminase .... **glutaminase**
glos/o- (pre) .... **gloss/o-**
glosipalatine arch ....
.... **glossopalatine arch**
glositis .... **glossitis**
glossafaringeal nerve ....
.... **glossopharyngeal nerve**
glotis .... **glottis**
Glowber's salt .... **Glauber's salt**
glowcoma .... **glaucoma**
gluckose tolerance test ....
.... **glucose tolerance test**
gluecagon .... **glucagon**
glueten .... **gluten****
glutinn .... **glutin****
glutraldehyde .... **glutaraldehyde**
gluttamic acid .... **glutamic acid**

gluttenin .... **glutenin**
glutus .... **gluteus**
glyal cells .... **glial cells**
glycashuria .... **glycosuria**
glyceen .... **glycine****
glycollipid .... **glycolipid**
glycollitic fast fibers ....
.... **glycolytic fast fibers**
glyco-protein .... **glycoprotein**
glycrogelatin .... **glycerogelatin**
glykogen .... **glycogen**
glyoma .... **glioma**
Glyseen .... **Glycine****
glyserite .... **glycerite**
gnawsheated .... **nauseated**
goaled therapy .... **gold therapy**
goenadatropin .... **gonadotropin**
goldstone .... **gallstone**
golgy apparatus .... **Golgi apparatus**
Gollgi tendon organs ....
.... **Golgi tendon organs**
gommer .... **gomer**
gonadd .... **gonad**
gonakoccus .... **gonococcus**
goneon .... **gonion****
gonerea .... **gonorrhea**
goneum .... **gonium****
gonn/o- (pre) .... **gon/o-**
gonnadotropin releasing
hormone ....
.... **gonadotropin releasing
hormone**
gonnococal urethritis ....
.... **gonococcal urethritis**
goolose .... **gulose**
goosbumps .... **goose bumps**
gooss flesh .... **goose flesh**
Goucher .... **Gaucher**
Gowcher disease ....
.... **Gaucher's disease**
gowt .... **gout**
goyter .... **goiter**
gp .... **GP**
-graf (suff) .... **-graph**
Graffenberg spot ..... **Grafenberg spot**
-graffy (suff) .... **-graphy**

Grafian follicle	**graafian follicle**	gripp	**grippe****
gram-pozitive bacteria		grizofulvin	**griseofulvin**
....	**gram-positive bacteria**	groath hormone	**growth hormone**
gramm	**gram****	groop insurance	**group insurance**
Gramm	**Gram****	groth	**growth**
-gramm (suff)	-gram	groupp practice	**group practice**
gramm/o- (pre)	**gram/o-**	grownd substance	
grammicidin	**gramicidin**	....	**ground substance**
gramm-negative bacteria		groyn	**groin**
....	**gram-negative bacteria**	GTT	**gtt.**
granaloma	**granuloma**	guiac test	**guaiac test**
granmal	**grand mal**	gulet	**gullet**
grannulocyte	**granulocyte**	gumm	**gum**
grannyala	**granula****	gurm	**germ**
grannyeler	**granular****	gurmicidal soap	**germicidal soap**
granyool	**granule****	Gutmaker Institute	
granyular endoplasmic reticulum		....	**Guttmacher Institute**
... **granular endoplasmic reticulum**		gutt	**gut****
grater curvature	**greater curvature**	Guyan-Baray	**Guillain-Barré**
graves disease	**Graves' disease**	gwanine	**guanine**
graype sugar	**grape sugar**	gygantism	**gigantism**
grey market	**gray market**	gynicology	**gynecology**
grey mater	**gray matter**	gynnek/o- (pre)	**gynec/o-**

H

habbit	**habit****	hard attack	**heart attack**
haf-life	**half-life**	hard pallate	**hard palate**
hailocaine	**halocaine**	harred of hearing	**hard of hearing**
hairlip	**harelip**	hart	**heart****
hakking	**hacking**	harte defects	**heart defects**
halatosis	**halitosis**	hart-lung machine	
haloosinogen	**hallucinogen**	....	**heart-lung machine**
halucination	**hallucination**	hasheesh	**hashish**
halusinate	**hallucinate**	Havversian canals	
halux	**hallux**	....	**Haversian canals**
hamertoe	**hammertoe**	hawmone	**hormone**
hammate	**hamate**	hawnch	**haunch****
hammstring	**hamstring**	hayr	**hair**
handikapped	**handicapped**	headake powder	**headache powder**
handycap	**handicap**	head stroke	**heatstroke**
hangnale	**hangnail**	heall	**heal****
hang ovver	**hangover**	health faslity	**health facility**
hannd	**hand**	health mantnance organization	
Hannsen	**Hansen****	....	**health maintenance**
Hansons disease	**Hansen's disease**		**organization**
haployd̥y	**haploidy**	hearr	**hear****
happloid	**haploid**	heart beet	**heartbeat**

Incorrect	Correct	Incorrect	Correct
heartbern	**heartburn**	hemoestaysis	**hemostasis**
heart-falure	**heart failure**	hemofilia	**hemophilia****
heart-mermer	**heart murmur**	hemogenius	**hemogeneous****
heat-prustation	**heat prostration**	hemorage	**hemorrhage****
Hechst-Roossel	**Hoechst-Roussel**	hemosstatiks	**hemostatics**
hedache	**headache**	hemotysis	**hemoptysis**
hedenism	**hedonism**	hempp	**hemp**
heebphrenia	**hebephrenia**	hemycardea	**hemicardia**
heeleotropic	**heliotropic**	hemyzigous	**hemizygous**
heeler	**healer**	hennbane	**henbane**
heelium	**helium**	Hennsen	**Hensen****
heelix	**helix**	hepetektomy	**hepatectomy**
heell .	**heel****	hepetitis	**hepatitis**
heema- (pre)	**hema-**	hepititus b	**hepatitis B**
heematinics	**hematinics**	heppat/o- (pre)	**hepat/o-**
heemattofagus	**hematophagous****	heppatic	**hepatic**
-heemea (suff)	**-hemia**	hepped/o- (pre)	**hept/o-**
heemo- (pre)	**hemo-**	heprin	**heparin**
heet exhaustion	**heat exhaustion**	Herb's palsy	**Erb's palsy**
heeting-pad	**heating pad**	heredditty	**heredity**
heir follicle	**hair follicle**	heredetery defect	**hereditary defect**
heksaklorophene	**hexachlorophene**	hernea	**hernia**
helkoprotein	**helicoprotein**	herpeas soster	**herpes zoster**
hellbone	**heel bone**	herpees	**herpes**
hellmint/o- (pre)	**helminth/o-**	herreditary	**hereditary**
hellper t cell	**helper T cell**	herroin	**heroin**
hellth insurance	**health insurance**	herrpes simplex	**herpes simplex**
helmentholigy	**helminthology**	hersutism	**hirsutism**
helth adminstrator		hete lamp	**heat lamp**
	health administrator	heteronimus	**heteronymous****
Helth Cair Financing		hetrologous	**heterologous****
Administration	**Health Care**	hetrovakksine therapy	
	Financing Administration		**heterovaccine therapy**
hemaglobbin	**hemoglobin**	hetterotropia	**heterotropia****
hematherepy	**hemotherapy**	hettr/o- (pre)	**hetero-**
hemattocritt test	**hematocrit test**	hettronomis	**heteronomous****
hemepplegia	**hemiplegia**	hewe	**hue**
hemeroids	**hemorrhoids**	hexxose sugar	**hexose sugar**
hemesfere	**hemisphere**	hey fever	**hay fever**
hemestassis	**hemostasis**	hi/o- (pre)	**hy/o-**
hemetollogy	**hematology**	hial/o- (pre)	**hyal/o-**
hemetoughagous	**hematophagus****	hi blood pressure	
hemitoma	**hematoma****		**high blood pressure**
hemm/i/o- (pre)	**hemi/o-**	hickup	**hiccup**
hemmastat	**hemostat**	hiddr/o/- (pre)	**hidr/o-**
hemmat/o- (pre)	**hemat/o-**	hiderate	**hydrate**
hemmatic	**hematic**	hiderofobia	**hydrophobia**
hemmofilus	**hemophilus**	hiderotherepy	**hydrotherapy**
hemoedyalisis	**hemodialysis**	hidrasteen	**hydrastine****

Incorrect	Correct	Incorrect	Correct
hidro- (pre)	**hydr/o**	hips/o- (pre)	**hyps/o-**
hidrocele	**hydrocele**	hisst/o- (pre)	**hist/o-**
hidrollisis	**hydrolysis**	hisster/o- (pre)	**hyster/o-**
hidroxxydehydrocorticosterone		hissteria	**hysteria**
	hydroxydehydrocorticosterone	hisstidine	**histidine**
Hiemlich maneuever		hisstory	**history**
	Heimlich maneuver	histacommpatibility antigens	
higeen	**hygiene**		**histocompatability antigens**
highdroxydezoxycorticosterone		histammine h	**histomine H**
	hydroxydesoxycorticosterone	histaplazmosis	**histoplasmosis**
highoid	**hyoid**	histerectomy	**hysterectomy**
highpermotility	**hypermotility**	histimeen	**histamine**
highpotention	**hypotension****	histollogy	**histology**
high-tuch product		histryonic personality	
	high-touch product		**histrionic personality**
himanjioma	**hemangioma**	hitadid mole	**hydadid mole**
himen	**hymen**	HIV antebody seeropositivity	
himolysis	**hemolysis**		**HIV antibodyseropositivity**
hinje joint	**hinge joint**	hiv antibody seronegativity	
hipe- (pre)	**hyp-**		**HIV antibody seronegativity**
hiper- (pre)	**hyper-**	HIV assimptomaticity	
hiperbaric chamber			**HIV asymptomaticity**
	hyperbaric chamber	HIV dezease	**HIV disease**
hiperkolesterolemia		hiztone	**histone****
	hypercholesterolemia**	hmo	**HMO**
hiperthalamic/o- (pre)		Hodjkins disease	
	hypothalamic/o		**Hodgkin's disease****
hipertonic solution		Hofman-Laroche	
	hypertonic solution		**Hoffman-La Roche**
hip joynt	**hip joint**	holacrine	**holocrine**
hipn/o- (pre)	**hypn/o-**	hole blood	**whole blood**
hipnosis	**hypnosis**	holeism	**holism**
hipnotonic solution		holenzyme	**holoenzyme**
	hypotonic solution	holisstic health	**holistic health**
hipo- (pre)	**hypo-**	holistic heeling	**holistic healing**
hipochondrium	**hypochondrium**	holistik medsin	**holistic medicine**
hipocratic oath	**Hippocratic oath**	holl/o- (pre)	**hol/o-**
hipodermic siringe		hollicrine gland	**holocrine gland**
	hypodermic syringe	hollistic approach	**holistic approach**
hipokolesteremia		hollocrine secretion	
	hypocholesterolemia		**holocrine secretion**
hipollipidemics	**hypolipidemia**	holow	**hollow**
hipothalim/o- (pre)	**hypothalam/o-**	homasexule	**homosexual**
hipoxia	**hypoxia**	homasistene	**homocysteine****
hipp bone	**hipbone**	homiopithy	**homeopathy**
hipperglicemia	**hyperglycemia****	homisside	**homicide**
hippnotics	**hypnotics**	hommi- (pre)	**home/o-**
hiprapolarization	**hyperpolarization**	homm/o- (pre)	**hom/o-**

Incorrect	Correct	Incorrect	Correct
hommologous	homologous**	humun t-cell lymphocyte virus	
hommosysteen	homocystine**		... human T-cell lymphocyte virus
homoeerotick	homoerotic	hunnchback	hunchback
homoll/o- (pre)	homol/o-	huntington's korea	
homostasis	homeostasis		Huntington's chorea
homozigot	homozygote	hurbal remidies	herbal remedies
homyopath	homeopath	hurmafrodite	hermaphrodite
honymoon sistitis		hurniated disc	herniated disk
	honeymoon cystitis	hurpes jenitalis	herpes genitalis
hookwurm	hookworm	hyatus	hiatus
hooping cough	whooping cough	hy-density lipoprotein	
horesontal	horizontal		high-density lipoprotein
hormoan replacement therapy		hyder/o- (pre)	hydr/o-
	hormone replacement therapy	hyderokloric acid	
horney layer	horny layer		hydrochloric acid
hornyhost surrogate		hydrasephalus	hydrocephalus
	Horneyhost surrogate	hydrasstatic pressure	
horpilation	horripilation		hydrostatic pressure
horrmonil therapy		hydrijen peroxide	
	hormonal therapy		hydrogen peroxide
horss	hoarse	hydroksycorticosterone	
hospitilazation	hospitalization		hydroxycorticosterone
hospitle bed	hospital bed	hydrosteneen	hydrastinine**
hospittal administrator		hyedro- (pre)	hydr/o-
	hospital administrator	Hymlich manoover	
hosspice	hospice		Heimlich maneuver
hosspital	hospital	hyoescyamus	hyoscyamus
hott flashes	hot flashes	hypadurmic needle	
housmaids knee	housemaid's knee		hypodermic needle
howlow	hollow	hypaklorous acid	
howse call	house call		hypochlorous acid
huemer/o- (pre)	humer/o-	hypakondrium	hyperchondrium
humain	humane**	hypamotility	hypomotility
humback	humpback	hyparopia	hyperopia
humer	humor	hypathurmia	hypothermia**
humerral	humeral**	hypeglossal	hypoglossal
humerral immunity		hypenefroma	hypernephroma
	humoral immunity	hyperdermic	hypodermic
humin	human**	hyperomanic personality	
humin korionic gonadotrophin			hypomanic personality
	human chorionic gonadotropin	hyperractive child syndrome	
huminnistic sychology			hyperactive child syndrome
	humanistic psychology	hyperrasidity	hyperacidity
hummer/o- (pre)	humer/o-	hyperrbaric oxegenation therapy	
hummyalin	humulin**		hyperbaric oxygenation therapy
humorrel	humoral**	hyperrimia	hyperemia
humorus	humerus**	hyperrinsulinism	hyperinsulinism
humulleen	humulene**	hyperrplazia	hyperplasia

Incorrect	Correct	Incorrect	Correct

hyperrthermia .... **hyperthermia****
hypesensitivity .... **hypersensitivity**
hypiglosal nerve ... **hypoglossal nerve**
hypiplazia .... **hypoplasia**
hypitrofy .... **hypertrophy**
hypnottic .... **hypnotic**
hypobaric therapy ....
.... **hyperbaric therapy**
hypoeglycemia .... **hypoglycemia****
hypofagia .... **hyperphagia**
hypokondria .... **hypochondria**
hypopraksia .... **hypopraxia**
hyposspadyis .... **hypospadias**

hypothiroydism .... **hypothyroidism**
hypoxxic hypoxxia .. **hypoxic hypoxia**
hypperventilation ..... **hyperventilation**
hypthalmus .... **hypothalamus**
hysterrical pursonality ....
.... **hysterical personality**
hysycamine .... **hyoscyamine**
hyue .... **hue**
hyuman imunodeficiency virus ....
.. **human immunodeficiency virus**
hyumid .... **humid**
hyves .... **hives**

I

-iak (suff) .... **-iac**
iatrajenic .... **iatrogenic**
-iatree (suff) .... **-iatry**
-iatrick (suff) .... **-iatric**
iattro- (pre) .... **iatro-**
ibaprofen .... **ibuprofen**
ice/o- (pre) .... **is/o-**
iceotonic contraction ....
.... **isotonic contraction**
ichihara test .... **Ishihara test**
iching .... **itching**
-ick (suff) .... **-ic**
ickter/o- (pre) .... **icter/o-**
ickthulin .... **ichthulin**
ickthy/o- (pre) .... **ichthy/o-**
ictheosis .... **ichthyosis**
icu .... **ICU**
idd .... **id****
-idda (suff) .... **-ida**
-iddea (suff) .... **-idea**
iddeo- (pre) .... **ideo-**
iddio- (pre) .... **idio-**
-iddrosis (suff) .... **-idrosis**
-ide (suff) .... **-id**
ideopathic .... **idiopathic**
ideot .... **idiot**
idine .... **iodine**
idoform .... **iodoform**
idyocy .... **idiocy**
iern .... **iron****
ilectromyograph ...... **electromyograph**

ileeytis .... **ileitis**
ileim .... **ileum****
ill- (pre) .... **il-**
ille/o- (pre) .... **ile/o-**
illeac .... **ileac****
illectuary .... **electuary**
illium .... **ilium****
illy/o- (pre) .... **ili/o-**
illyostomy .... **ileostomy**
ilness .... **illness**
ilusion .... **illusion**
ilyak .... **iliac****
imerse .... **immerse**
imiturity reaction ....
.... **immaturity reaction**
imm- (pre) .... **im-**
immergency .... **emergency**
immipramine .... **imipramine**
immplantation .... **implantation**
immunechemistry ....
.... **immunochemistry**
immunesupressent ....
.... **immunosuppressant**
immunnoglobulin ....**immunoglobulin**
immunoesurpressives ....
.... **immunosuppressives**
immyanization .... **immunization**
immyoonity .... **immunity**
imparement .... **impairment**
impatence .... **impotence**
imperegnation .... **impregnation**

40

Incorrect	Correct
impitigo	impetigo
impullse	impulse
imune responses	immune responses
imunetherapy	immunotherapy
imunization therapy	immunization therapy
imuno- (pre)	immuno-
imyune therapy	immune therapy
inatropic agent	inotropic agent
inbalance	in balance**
inballanse	imbalance**
inbawn immunity	inborn immunity
incadents	incidents
incission and drainage	incision and drainage
incurible	incurable
incyubation period	incubation period
indakation	indication
indaspozed	indisposed
indeependent practice association	independent practice association
indegestion	indigestion
indexx finger	index finger
indiann hemp	Indian hemp
indivviddual psychology	individual psychology
indoosed abortion	induced abortion
industreal psychology	industrial psychology
ineebreated	inebriated
iner ear	inner ear
inerrvate	innervate**
infanntalism	infantilism
infar- (pre)	infra-**
infared therapy	infrared therapy
infarktion	infarction**
infecshous	infectious
infeerior	inferior
infekt	infect
infektion	infection
infermary	infirmary
inferr- (pre)	infer-**
infesstation	infestation
infilltrative	infiltrative

Incorrect	Correct
infint	infant
infintyle paralysis	infantile paralysis
infireority complex	inferiority complex
inflaimed	inflamed
inflimation	inflammation
influwenza	influenza
infurm	infirm
infurtility	infertility
infyusion pump	infusion pump
ingection	injection
ingreediant	ingredient
ingroan toenail	ingrown toenail
inhailant	inhalant
inhallation	inhalation
inhilator	inhalator**
injekt	inject
injery	injury
inkapacity	incapacity
inkompitent	incompetent
inkrust	incrust**
inkus	incus
inkyubater	incubator
inmunology	immunology
inn- (pre)	in-
innactive	inactive
innborn era of metabolism	inborn error of metabolism
inncizura	incisura**
inncompatable	incompatible
inncompleet	incomplete
inncontinence	incontinence
innert	inert
innextreemis	in extremis
innfectious dizease	infectious disease
innflate	inflate
innhale	inhale
innitial	initial
innkwest	inquest
inno- (pre)	ino-
innoculation	inoculation
innsanity	insanity
inn situ	in situ
innstep	instep
innsult	insult
innter- (pre)	inter-**

Incorrect	Correct	Incorrect	Correct
inntern	interne**	interfase	interphase**
inntestin/o- (pre)	intestin/o-	intermuscular	intramuscular
inntestinal gas	intestinal gas	internel medecine	internal medicine
inntoksicant	intoxicant	internuron	interneuron
inntolrance	intolerance	interocrinin	enterocronin
inntra- (pre)	intra-**	interogastrone	enterogastrone
inntrinsic clotting pathway	intrinsic clotting pathway	interrmedin	intermedin
inntro- (pre)	intro-	interrnal enviroment	internal environment
inn utero	in utero	interrnunsial neuron	internuncial neuron
inn vitro fertilization	in vitro fertilization	interselular fluid	intercellular fluid
inocus	innocuous	interventrickuler	intraventricular**
inomminate artery	innominate artery	interversion	introversion
inpashent	inpatient**	intesstinal obstruction	intestinal obstruction
inplant	implant	intestenal mucose	intestinal mucose
insecteside	insecticide	intestinn	intestine
insemmination	insemination	intevenntricler	interventricular**
insest	incest	intevention	intervention
insidense	incidence	intevenus	intravenous**
insillinase	insulinase	intireor	interior
insipient	incipient	intra-abdominal abscesses	inter-abdominal abscesses
insision	incision	intracostal nerve	intercostal nerve
insizher	incisure**	intrajection	introjection**
insomia	insomnia	intramediary	intermediary
insparation	inspiration	intramission	intromission**
insperater	inspirator	intrapose	interpose
inspratory reserve volume	inspiratory reserve volume	intrastitial cells	interstitial cells
instibility	instability	intravvert	introvert
instink	instinct	introvenous infusion	intravenous infusion
instrament	instrument	intruterine devise	intrauterine device
insufishent	insufficient	inturn	intern**
insurts	inserts	inturnal cuniform	internal cuneiform
insyalin	insulin	inturnist	internist
insysor	incisor**	invatase	invertase
intacourse	intercourse	inveetro	in vitro
intafase	interface**	invilid	invalid
intafereon	interferon	invilutional sychosis	involutional psychosis
intamission	intermission**	involintary muscle	involuntary muscle
intarmitent	intermittent		
intavenous	intervenous**		
integgumentery system	integumentary system		
intennsive care unit	intensive care unit		
intercorse	intercourse		

42

invurtibrate .... **invertebrate**
iodifors .... **iodophors**
ipicack .... **ipecac**
ippecacwana .... **ipecacuanha**
iradiation .... **irradiation**
iredektomy .... **iridectomy****
iregularity .... **irregularity**
iremeable .... **irremeable****
iremeediable .... **irremediable****
irigate .... **irrigate**
irin lung .... **iron lung**
iritibility .... **irritability**
iritible bowl syndrome ....
.... **irritable bowel syndrome**
irr- (pre) .... **ir-**
irrid/o- (pre) .... **irid/o-**
irriversable .... **irreversible**
iruption .... **eruption**
isalation .... **isolation**
isametric contraction ....
.... **isometric contraction**
isapropil .... **isopropyl**
isatonnic exercise .... **isotonic exercise**
isekromosome .... **isochromosome**
ise pac .... **ice pack**
ishi/o- (pre) .... **ischi/o-**
ishomenia .... **ischomenia**

isillation chamber ....
.... **isolation chamber**
-isis (suff) .... **-iasis**
isitonic solution .... **isotonic solution**
iskemia .... **ischemia**
iskeum .... **ischium**
ismus of the uterine cavity ....
...... **isthmus of the uterine cavity**
isoemetrick exercise ....
.... **isometric exercise**
isollucine .... **isoleucine**
isonazid .... **isoniazid**
-isst (suff) .... **-ist**
-itte (suff) .... **-ite**
-ittic (suff) .... **-itic**
iud .... **IUD**
iv .... **IV**
ivee pole .... **ivy pole**
ivy needle .... **IV needle**
-ix (suff) .... **-ics**
iyewash .... **eyewash**
-iyim (suff) .... **-ium**
iyinizing .... **ionizing**
iyodide .... **iodide**
iyulio- (pre) .... **iulio-**
-izm (suff) .... **-ism**

J

Jacob-Kreutzfeldt ....
.... **Jakob-Creutzfeldt**
jallop .... **jalap**
Jannsen .... **Jansen****
jawndice .... **jaundice**
jeen pool .... **gene pool**
jegunum .... **jejunum**
jejoon/o- (pre) .... **jejun/o-**
jel-filled implant .... **gel-filled implant**
jell .... **gel**
jellys .... **jellies**
jen- (pre) .... **gen-**
jender dysphoria .... **gender dysphoria**
jene frequency .... **gene frequency**
jeneral medicine .... **general medicine**

jeneric-name drug ....
.... **generic-name drug**
jenesial stage .... **genesial stage**
jenesis .... **genesis**
jenetic code .... **genetic code**
jenital .... **genital****
jenitals .... **genitals**
jenito-urinary .... **genitourinary**
Jennsen .... **Jensen****
jeno- (pre) .... **geno-**
jenome .... **genome**
jeraneal .... **geraniol****
jeriatrics .... **geriatrics**
jermacide .... **germicide**
jerman measles .... **German measles**

Incorrect	Correct	Incorrect	Correct
jestation	gestation	Jonson & Jonson	
jett lag	jet lag		Johnson & Johnson
jimsin weed	jimsonweed	Joungian psychology	
jingivitis	gingivitis		Jungian psychology
jinjiv/o- (pre)	gingiv/o-	joynt disease	joint disease
jones	Jones	juggular trunk	jugular trunk

K

Incorrect	Correct	Incorrect	Correct
Kagel exercises	Kegel exercises	kari/o- (pre)	kary/o-
kalcium	calcium	karina	carina
kalendar rhythm	calendar rhythm	karititis	keratitis
kalla-azar	kala-azar	karitype	karyotype
kallus	callus**	karotid	carotid**
kalomel	calomel	karpal	carpal
kalyx	calyx**	karpus	carpus
kancrum	cancrum	kartilage	cartilage
Kandida albicans	Candida albicans	kascara	cascara
Kandidial vaginitis		kase	case
	candidal vaginitis	kaseenogen	caseinogen
kandy stripper	candy striper	kast	cast
kanine	canine	katalepsy	catalepsy
Kann	Kahn	kataplexy	cataplexy
Kannimicin	Kanamycin	katatonia	catatonia
kannula	cannula	kath- (pre)	cath-
kantharides	cantharides	kathartic	cathartic
kapillary network		katheterization	catheterization
	capillary network	Katocis	ketosis**
kapitation fee	capitation fee	katonia	catatonia
Kapossi sarcoma	Kaposi's sarcoma	kavity	cavity
kaput	caput	Kay Y jelly	KY jelly
karacter disorder		kemecal stimulation of the brain	
	character disorder		chemical stimulation of the brain
karatid-body chemorecptor		kemical dependency	
	carotid-body chemoreceptor		chemical dependency
karbohydrase	carbohydrase	kemosynthesis	chemosynthesis
karbon	carbon	kemotherapy	chemotherapy
karboxy peptidase		-keneesis (suff)	-kinesis
	carboxypeptidase	kenesi/o- (pre)	kinesi/o-
karbuncle	carbuncle**	kenetic	kinetic
kardeograph	cardiograph	kerataplasty	keratoplasty
kardiac arrest	cardiac arrest	keretitis	keratitis
kardiack muscle	cardiac muscle	keretolitics	keratolytics
kardiotherapy	cardiotherapy	keritosis	keratosis**
karditis	carditis		

44

kerrat/o- (pre) .... **kerat/o-**
kerratin .... **keratin**
kerratoma .... **keratoma**
ketoe- (pre) .... **keto-**
kettone .... **ketone**
kideny basin .... **kidney basin**
kidnee .... **kidney**
kidnystone .... **kidney stone**
kifosis .... **kyphosis**
killd-virus vaccine ....
.... **killed-virus vaccine**
kimagraf .... **kymograph**
kineesiology .... **kinesiology**
kini/o- (pre) .... **kin/e/o-**
kinises .... **kinesis**
kinnesthesia .... **kinesthesia**
kinnin .... **kinin**
kiro- (pre) .... **chiro-**
kiropody .... **chiropody**
kiroprakter .... **chiropractor**
kirurgical .... **chirurgical**
kising disease .... **kissing disease**
klamp .... **clamp**
klamydia .... **chlamydia**
klavicle .... **clavicle**
kleft palate .... **cleft palate**
klimatotherapy .... **climatotherapy**
klimax .... **climax**
klinic .... **clinic**
klinical medicine .... **clinical medicine**
klitoridectomy .... **clitoridectomy**
klone .... **clone**
kloral hydrate .... **chloral hydrate**
kloraplast .... **chloroplast**
klordiazepoxide ...... **chlordiazepoxide**
klorine .... **chlorine**
klosed panel practice ....
.... **closed panel practice**
klostridium .... **clostridium**
klot .... **clot**
klove oil .... **clove oil**
klubfoot .... **clubfoot**
kneebrace .... **knee brace**
kneeontology .... **neonatology**
kneoplastic .... **neoplastic**
knewmonitis .... **pneumonitis**
knewrogenic .... **neurogenic**

knight-eating syndrome ....
.... **night-eating syndrome**
knitt .... **nit**
knockshus .... **noxious**
knot-for-profit .... **not-for-profit**
knovocaine .... **novocaine**
knowdal .... **nodal**
koagulation .... **coagulation**
kobalt therapy .... **cobalt therapy**
koccidiodomycosis ....
.... **coccidioidomycosis**
koccigeal nerve .... **coccygeal nerve**
-koccus (suff) .... **-coccus**
koccyx .... **coccyx**
kochlear nerve .... **cochlear nerve**
kocklea .... **cochlea****
kodeine .... **codeine**
kognitive service .... **cognitive service**
kol- (pre) .... **col-**
kolecystectomy .... **cholecystectomy**
kolecystokinin .... **cholecystokinin**
koler .... **kola**
koleric .... **choleric****
kolesterol .... **cholesterol**
koli- (pre) .... **coli-**
kolicky pain .... **colicky pain**
kollagen injection ....
.... **collagen injection**
kolla nut .... **kola nut**
kollapsed lung .... **collapsed lung**
kolo- (pre) .... **colo-**
kolocynth .... **colocynth**
kolon .... **colon**
kolonic irrigation ... **colonic irrigation**
kolostomy .... **colostomy**
koma .... **coma**
komedo .... **comedo**
kommunity medicine ....
.... **community medicine**
kompensatory growth ....
.... **compensatory growth**
komplementary medicine ....
.... **complementary medicine**
kompulsive personality ....
.... **compulsive personality**
koncha .... **concha**
kondrio- (pre) .... **chondrio-**

kondrotrophic hormone .... **chondrotropic hormone**		Krebbs cycle .... **Krebs cycle**	
konducting system .... **conducting system**		krepitus .... **crepitus**	
kondylomata acuminata .... **condylomata acuminata**		kript- (pre) .... **crypt-**	
kone .... **cone**		kripto- (pre) .... **crypto-**	
kongestive heart failure .... **congestive heart failure**		kriptogenic .... **cryptogenic**	
konnective tissue disorders .... **connective tissue disorders**		kroloquine .... **chloroquine**	
konstitutional therapy .... **constitutional therapy**		kromatid .... **chromatid**	
kontact therapy .... **contact therapy**		kromosomal aberration .... **chromosomal aberration**	
kontamination .... **contamination**		kronic cystic mastitis .... **chronic cystic mastitis**	
kontractility .... **contractility**		krossing-over .... **crossing-over**	
kontraindication .... **contraindication**		kryobirth .... **cryobirth**	
konvergence insufficiency .... **convergence insufficiency**		kryonic suspension .... **cryonic suspension**	
konversion reaction .... **conversion reaction**		kryotherapy .... **cryotherapy**	
kopayment .... **co-payment**		*Kryptococcis neoformans* .... ***Cryptococcus neoformans***	
kopr- (pre) .... **copr-**		kuack .... **quack**	
kopro- (pre) .... **copro-**		KUBB .... **KUB**	
koprolith .... **coprolith**		kuldoscopy .... **culdoscopy**	
koprophilia .... **coprophilia**		kulture .... **culture**	
koranary thrombosis .... **coronary thrombosis**		kuneiform .... **cuneiform**	
korea .... **chorea**		kurare .... **curare**	
korneal transplant .... **corneal transplant**		kusp .... **cusp**	
korn sugar .... **corn sugar**		kuspid .... **cuspid**	
koroid coat .... **choroid coat**		kwad- (pre) .... **quad-**	
koronary artery bypass graft .... **coronary artery bypass graft**		kwadriplegia .... **quadriplegia**	
koroo .... **koro**		kwality .... **quality**	
korpus luteum .... **corpus luteum**		Kwalude .... **Quaalude**	
korronary infraction .... **coronary infarction**		kwantitative .... **quantitative**	
korticko- (pre) .... **cortico-**		kwart .... **quart**	
korticosterone .... **corticosterone**		kwarten .... **quartan**	
kortisol .... **cortisol**		kwarter evil .... **quarter evil**	
kortisone .... **cortisone**		kwartz lamp .... **quartz lamp**	
Kottex .... **Kotex**		kwashiker .... **kwashiorkor**	
kotton swab .... **cotton swab**		Kwel .... **Kwell**	
koxa .... **coxa**		kwestionible .... **questionable**	
		kwietly .... **quietly**	
		kwinolones .... **quinolones**	
		kwinque .... **quinque****	
		kwoshent .... **quotient**	
		kwotidian ague .... **quotidian ague**	
		kwyescent .... **quiescent**	
		kwynine .... **quinine**	
		kymotrypsin .... **chymotrypsin**	

L

Incorrect	Correct
labbia majora	labia majora
labbile	labile**
labeal	labial**
labea minnora	labia minora
laber	labor
labered breething	labored breathing
labirinth	labyrinth
labratory technician	laboratory technician
labyum	labium
laccrim/o- (pre)	lacrim/o-
lackedalbumin	lactalbumin
lackramale	lacrimale**
lackrimal gland	lacrimal gland
lacktase	lactase
lacktoes	lactose
lackunar	lacunar**
lacoona	lacuna**
lacramal	lacrimal**
lactaferrous sinus	lactiferous sinus
lactajenic hormone	lactigenic hormone
lactial gland	lacteal gland
Ladelaw	Laidlaw
laffing gas	laughing gas
laid low	Laidlow
lakt/i/o- (pre)	lact/i/o-
laktation	lactation
laktic acid	lactic acid
lalech league	La Leche League
-lallia (suff)	-lalia
La Maze	Lamaze
lamena	laminar**
lamness	lameness
lammina	lamina**
lanalin	lanolin
lancit	lancet**
Langa	Lange**
Langans	Langhans**
Langehans	Langerhans**
langer	languor**
Langor	Langer**
langwishing	languishing
lansed	lanced**
lantse	lance
laparr/o- (pre)	lapar/o-
laperotomy pack	laparotomy pack
laporotomy	laparotomy
lappack	lap pack
lapparoscopy	laparoscopy
laringectomy	laryngectomy
larinx	larynx
larje intestine	large intestine
larringoscope	laryngoscope
larryng/o- (pre)	laryng/o-
laryndjitis	laryngitis
Lasa fever	Lassa fever
lasar therapy	laser therapy
lasatude	lassitude
lasseration	laceration
latinsy-lukoplakia	latency leukoplakia
latral inhibition	lateral inhibition
lattency	latency
latter/o- (pre)	later/o-
lattisimus dorsey	latissimus dorsi
lavvage	lavage
lawdanum	laudanum
lawrdosis	lordosis
laxitive	laxative
laybia	labia
laytent period	latent period
lazer	laser**
lazer surgery	laser surgery
lazzer	lazar**
leatch	leach**
leboyyer	Leboyer
lecthinase	lecithinase
Ledderle	Lederle
led poisoning	lead poisoning
leekage	leakage
leetch	leech**
leeter	liter**
leethal dose	lethal dose
lefhanded	left-handed

47

Incorrect	Correct	Incorrect	Correct
legementa	ligamenta**	liggand	ligand
legg	leg	liggiment	ligament**
lejinnaire's disease		ligiture	ligature
	legionnaires' disease	likesose	lyxose
lemen	lemon	likwid incense	liquid incense
lenns	lens	lim	limb
lentego	lentigo	limbis	limbus
leo- (pre)	lio-	lime disease	Lyme disease
lepera	lepra**	limf	lymph
leppedosperosis	leptospirosis	limfatic duck	lymphatic duct
lepper	leper**	limmbic system	limbic system
leppo- (pre)	lepo-	limmphatic drainage	
-leppsia (suff)	-lepsia		lymphatic drainage
-leppsis (suff)	-lepsis	limph/o- (pre)	lymph/o-
leppt/o- (pre)	lepto-	linaleeic	linoleic**
lepptandra	leptandra	linament	liniment
leprisy	leprosy	lineleenic	linolenic**
-lepsee (suff)	-lepsy	linfoma	lymphoma
leptaspira	leptospira	lingal papila	lingual papilae
lerning disabilities		lingg/i- (pre)	ling/i-
	learning disabilities	linggo- (pre)	lingo-
lesathoprotein	lecithoprotein	lingwal braces	lingual braces
lesbean	lesbian	lingwel	lingual**
leser curvature	lesser curvature	lingyala	lingula**
lesh	leche**	liniar	linear**
lessithin	lecithin	linkije	linkage
leukasite- (pre)	leukocyto-	linnea	linea**
leukasito- (pre)	leukocyto-	linnen	linen**
leukasitosis	leukocytosis	linnin	linin**
leukorea	leukorrhea	linolick	linolic**
levv/o- (pre)	lev/o-	linph-node	lymph node
levvel	level	linyae	lineae**
levvorfenol	levorphanol	lioh- (pre)	leio-
levvulose	levulose	lipakaic	lipocaic
-lexxia (suff)	-lexia	liper	lipa**
lezbian	lesbian	lipisuction	liposuction
lezion	lesion	lipoksidase	lipoxidase
libeedo	libido	lipomma	lipoma
libreum	Librium	lipp/o- (pre)	lip/o-
licin	lysin**	lippaoprotein	lipoprotein
licine	lycine**	lippase	lipase
lidd	lid	lipper	lippa**
lieo- (pre)	leio-	lippid	lipid
life-threttening	life-threatening	lipps	lips**
life-time maximum		liqwid	liquid
	lifetime maximum	lis- (pre)	lys-
liffe-support system		lisenced practical nurse	
	life-support system		licensed practical nurse

48

Incorrect	Correct	Incorrect	Correct

lisergic acid dyethylamide ....
.... **lysergic acid diethylamide**
-lisin (suff) .... **-lysin**
-lisis (suff) .... **-lysis**
liso- (pre) .... **lyso-**
lisosome .... **lysosome**
lissps .... **lisps****
-lite (suff)................................. **-lyte**
liteheadedness .... **lightheadedness**
litur .... **litter****
lithatripsy .... **lithotripsy**
-lithe (suff).................................. **-lith**
litheum carbonate ....
.... **lithium carbonate**
lithitrite .... **lithotrite**
lithottomy .... **lithotomy**
lithyum.................................. **lithium**
-litic (suff) .... **-lytic**
littel finger .... **little finger**
livirus-vaccine .... **live virus vaccine**
livver...................................... **liver****
livving well........................ **living will**
livvor...................................... **livor****
livvor spot........................... **liver spot**
loab ....**lobe**
lobb/i/o- (pre) .... **lob/i/o-**
lobis .... **lobus****
lo blood pressure ....
.... **low blood pressure**
lobottimy............................ **lobotomy**
lobyalie .... **lobuli****
lobyule .... **lobule****
lobz .... **lobes****
locamoshion .... **locomotion**
locjaw .... **lockjaw**
locle .... **local****
loe-density lipoprotein ....
.... **low-density lipoprotein**
logg/o- (pre) .... **log/o-**
-loggy (suff)............................... **-logy**
lo-grade fever .... **low-grade fever**
-lojist (suff).............................. **-logist**
lokal anesthetic .... **local anesthetic**
lokia ....**lochia**
lokial .... **lochial****
lokus .... **locus**
long cancer .... **lung cancer**
looce .... **loose****

Loo Gerrigs disease ....
.... **Lou Gehrig's disease**
lookocyte ....**leukocyte**
loomen .... **lumen**
loope .... **loop****
loopus .... **lupus**
loot- (pre) .... **lute-**
lootio- (pre) .... **luteo-**
losenge .... **lozenge**
lowse.. **louse**
lowwer-extremities ....
.... **lower extremities**
loyn .... **loin**
lpn .... **LPN**
lubracant .... **lubricant**
luc/o- (pre) .... **leuc/o-**
lucacyt/o- (pre) .... **leucocyt/o-**
lucine ....**leucine****
luek/o- (pre) .... **leuk/o-**
luekemia .... **leukemia**
luk/o- (pre) .... **leuc/o-**
luke/o- (pre) .... **leuk/o-**
lukine .... **leukin****
lukocyte/o- (pre) .... **leucocyt/o-**
lukopenia .... **leukopenia**
lumba vurtebrae .... **lumbar vertebrae**
lumbbar puncture .. **lumbar puncture**
lumber nerve .... **lumbar nerve**
lumenole ....**luminal****
luminil .... **Luminal****
lummb- (pre) ....**lumb-**
lummbago .... **lumbago**
lummbo- (pre) ....**lumbo-**
lummpektomy .... **lumpectomy**
lunbar nodes .... **lumbar nodes**
lung canser ....**lung cancer**
lung serfacant .... **lung surfactant**
lunng .... **lung**
lupe .... **loupe****
lupis erythematosus ....
.... **lupus erythematosus**
luppus vulgaris .... **lupus vulgaris**
luse.. **lues****
lutial phrase .... **luteal phase**
lutinizing hormone ....
.... **luteinizing hormone**
luvidity................................... **lividity**
ly .... **lye****

Incorrect	Correct	Incorrect	Correct
lyasol	lyosol**	lymphasyte	lymphocyte
lydocaine	lidocaine	lymphoyd tishue	lymphoid tissue
lyeseen	lysine**	lynfakine	lymphokine
Lyesoul	Lysol**	lynph gland	lymph gland
lymf	lymph	lysazime	lysozyme
lymfatic sistem	lymphatic system	lyseen	lysine**
lymphaddenopathy sindrome			
	lymphadenopathy syndrome		

M

Incorrect	Correct	Incorrect	Correct
macarocefelus	macrocephalus**	mail hypogonadism	
macerphage	macrophage		male hypgonadism
machuration	maturation	mail menopause	male menopause
machure	mature	maintinence	maintenance
machurity	maturity	maitenence	maintenance
mackr- (pre)	macr-	majer kalyx	major calyx
mackro- (pre)	macro-	majer sergery	major surgery
mackroprossopea	macroprosopy	makonium	meconium
mackrosefalous	macrocephalous**	makradaktily	macrodactyly**
macksimel	maximal	makrobiotic	macrobiotic
macksimum	maximum	makrodacktilia	macrodactylia**
mackyalar	macular**	makroscopic	macroscopic
macroeprosopea	macroprosopia	makula	macula**
macyule	macule**	malacklusion	malocclusion
mad-ditch	mad itch	malajusment	maladjustment
madiastinal	mediastinal	malak- (pre)	malac-
mad man	madman	malako- (pre)	malaco-
magganstrasse	Maganstrasse	malapsorption syndromes	
maggnesia	magnesia		malabsorption syndromes
maggnetic resenance imaging		malaryotherepy	malariatherapy
	magnetic resonance imaging	maleable	malleable
magnatic	magnetic	maledee	maladie**
magneesium oxide		malese	malaise
	magnesium oxide	malet finger	mallet finger
magneezium	magnesium	malette	mallet
magnezium hidroxide		malfermation	malformation
	magnesium hydroxide	malidy	malady**
magniseum citrate		malingring	malingering
	magnesium citrate	mall- (pre)	mal-
magor surgery	major surgery	mallabsorbtion	malabsorption
magot therapy	maggot therapy	mallan- (pre)	melan-
mailayze	malaise	mallarea	malaria**
mail climacteric	male climacteric	-mallasia (suff)	-malacia

50

Incorrect	Correct	Incorrect	Correct
malle	**mal****	mantell	**mantle**
malled sugar	**malt sugar**	manuver	**manoeuver**
maller	**malar**	manya	**mania**
mallfunction	**malfunction**	manyuel	**manual**
mallignancy	**malignancy**	mapel sugar	**maple sugar**
mallignent coytal headaches		marawana	**marijuana**
	malignant coital headaches	margoe	**margo**
mallpractise	**malpractice**	marjin	**margin**
malnootrition	**malnutrition**	marow cavity	**marrow cavity**
malpraktiss insurance		marrginel	**marginal**
	malpractice insurance	marroe	**marrow**
maltace	**maltase****	marterdum	**martyrdom**
malyus	**malleus**	mas	**mass**
mam- (pre)	**mamm-**	masage	**massage****
mama	**mamma**	masakism	**masochism**
mama- (pre)	**mamma-**	maseration	**maceration**
mamatropic hormone		maseter	**masseter**
	mammotropic hormone	masheen	**machine**
mami- (pre)	**mammi-**	masive	**massive**
maming	**maiming**	masking off simptoms	
mammery gland	**mammary gland**		**masking of symptoms**
mammiplasty	**mammoplasty**	maskuline	**masculine**
mamo- (pre)	**mammo-**	mass cell	**mast cell**
mamografee	**mammography**	massed/o- (pre)	**mast/o-**
mamogramme	**mammogram**	massif bleeding	**massive bleeding**
Man	**Mann****	massk of pregnency	
mandable	**mandible**		**mask of pregnancy**
-manea (suff)	**-mania**	masstektimy	**mastectomy**
manestreaming	**mainstreaming**	massterplastea	**mastoplastia****
manijed care	**managed care**	masster too-step test	
maninjeal	**meningeal**		**master two-step test**
manje	**mange**	-masstia (suff)	**-mastia**
mann	**man****	masstoid prosess	**mastoid process**
manndibuler	**mandibular**	masstosstomy	**mastostomy****
manndibuler nerve		mastaplassia	**mastoplasia****
	mandibular nerve	masterbation	**masturbation**
manndrell	**mandrel****	mastidecktomy	**mastoidectomy**
mann drill	**mandril****	mastittis	**mastitis**
mannic depression		mastottany	**mastotomy****
	manic depression	mastoyd	**mastoid**
mannipilation	**manipulation**	mast sell stabalizers	
mannometer	**manometer**		**mast cell stabilizers**
mannuel	**manual**	matchure	**mature**
manoc-depresive sychosis		matereal	**material****
	manic-depressive psychosis	material medica	**materia medica**
manoobrium	**manubrium**	matirea	**materia****
manoover	**manoeuver**	matoority	**maturity**
manoze	**manose**	matour	**mature**

Incorrect	Correct	Incorrect	Correct
matress	**mattress**	meedi- (pre)	**medi-**
matricks	**matrix**	meedial	**medial**
matternity	**maternity**	meedian cubital vein	
maturnity hospital			**median cubital vein**
	maternity hospital	meedio- (pre)	**medio-**
-mawfy (suff)	**-morphy**	meedium	**medium**
Mawl	**Mall****	Meed-Johnson	**Mead-Johnson**
mawltose	**maltose****	meel	**meal**
maxallery nerve	**maxillary nerve**	meen	**mean**
maxila	**maxilla**	meetus	**meatus**
mayjor medical	**major medical**	meezles	**measles****
mayl	**male**	meezly	**measly****
mayler	**malar**	megaloppsee	**megalopsia****
Maylox	**Maalox**	megecaryocite	**megakaryocyte**
-maynia (suff)	**-mania**	-megelly (suff)	**-megaly**
Maynière's syndrome		megelomannic	**megalomanic****
	Ménière's syndrome	meggal- (pre)	**megal-**
mayter	**mater**	meggalo- (pre)	**megalo-**
mayutic	**maieutic**	megilopea	**megalopia****
mazer	**maser**	meglomaniak	**megalomaniac****
Mazlow	**Maslow**	mekanical heart	**mechanical heart**
md	**MD**	mekinism	**mechanism**
meadia	**media**	melazma	**melasma**
meaningococcal	**meningococcal**	melencolic	**melancholic**
meazle	**measle****	meletonin	**melatonin**
meche	**mesh**	melinin	**melanin**
mechinoresepter	**mechanoreceptor**	melinkolia	**melancholia****
mecurichrome	**Mercurochrome**	melinoma	**melanoma**
medacare	**Medicare**	mellanasyte	**melanocyte**
medacation	**medication**	mellanin	**melanin**
meddacated dressing		mellankolea	**melancholiac****
	medicated dressing	mellano- (pre)	**melan/o-**
meddecate	**medicate****	mellencholic	**melancholic****
meddian	**median**	mellenoma	**melanoma**
meddic	**medic**	mellibyose	**melibiose**
meddicine	**medicine**	*mellisa*	*Melissa*
meddula	**medulla**	membrayna	**membrana****
medean nerve	**median nerve**	membraynus	**membranous**
medeated transport		memmbrain	**membrane****
	mediated transport	memry cell	**memory cell**
medecaid	**Medicaid****	menapaws	**menopause**
medellery	**medullary**	menark	**menarche**
medicil examiner		menarky	**menarche**
	medical examiner	Mendle	**Mendel**
medicly indijent	**medically indigent**	meneng- (pre)	**mening-**
medikal inshurance		menengi- (pre)	**meningi-**
	medical insurance	menengo- (pre)	**meningo-**
Medlers	**MEDLARS**	menenjitis	**meningitis**

Incorrect	Correct	Incorrect	Correct
menepausel	**menopausal**	mesethilioma	**mesothelioma**
meneragia	**menorrhagia**	meshure	**measure**
menincks	**meninx**	meskalin	**mescaline**
meninks	**meninx**	mesquito	**mosquito**
menistration	**menstruation****	mess/o- (pre)	**mes/o-**
menn- (pre)	**men-**	messatapelic	**mesatipellic****
mennacme	menacme	messathelea	**mesothelia****
Menndilean laws	**mendelian laws**	messcal	**mescal**
mennexenia	**menoxenia**	messetipelvik	**mesatipelvic**
mennings	**meninges**	messinjer RNA	**messenger RNA**
menninjioma	**meningioma**	messoglea	**mesoglea****
menniskus	**meniscus**	messothilyal	**mesothelial****
menno- (pre)	**meno-**	messovaryan	**mesovarian****
mennostatus	menostatis	metabilism	**metabolism**
mennstrual extraction		metabollic rate	**metabolic rate**
....	**menstrual extraction**	metacarpo- (pre)	**metacarpo-**
menntal hygene	**mental hygiene**	metafase	metaphase
mennthol	**menthol****	metakarpel	**metacarpal**
mensees	menses	metapeum	**metopium****
menstral migraine		metastisize	**metastasize**
....	**menstrual migraine**	metasychology	**metapsychology**
menstruel flucks	**menstrual flux**	metebolic alcalosis	
menstrule cycle	**menstrual cycle**	....	**metabolic alkalosis**
mentel hospital	**mental hospital**	metecarp- (pre)	**metacarp-**
menthalatum	**Mentholatum**	metecromasee	metachromasia
menthil	**menthyl****	metemorfoze	**metamorphose****
mentil retardation		meteprotien	**metaprotein**
....	**mental retardation**	meter- (pre)	**metr-**
mentin	**menton**	meternal	**maternal**
mentiside	**menticide**	metero- (pre)	**metro-**
mentle illness	**mental illness**	meteropeksia	**metropexia****
mently	**mentally**	*metesoa*	*Metazoa***
meperobimate	**meprobamate**	metetars- (pre)	**metatars-**
mepezeen	mepazine	metetarsall	metatarsal
mepperidine	**meperidine**	metetarso- (pre)	**metatarso-**
meracrin	**merocrine**	methamfetamin hydroclorate	
mercurric cloride		....	**methamphetamine hydrochlorate**
....	**mercuric chloride**	methannall	methanal**
mercurrus chloride		methedology	**methodology**
....	**mercurous chloride**	methedon	**methadone**
merkyurial ointment		methedrine	Methedrine
....	**mercurial ointment**	metheen	**methene****
mermer	**murmur**	methein	**methine****
merrbrominn	**merbromin**	methenol	methanol**
merrocrine gland	**merocrine gland**	methid	**method**
mesadurm	**mesoderm**	methil	**methyl**
mesage	**message****	methilene blue	**methylene blue**
mesavaryum	**mesovarium****		

Incorrect	Correct	Incorrect	Correct
Methiolate	Merthiolate	micomicin	mycomycin
methisilin	methicillin	micossis	mycosis
methynine	methionine	micotic	mycotic
metibolick	metabolic	micrabioligy	microbiology
metimeer	metamere**	micrascope	microscope
metiplazia	metaplasia	micratubull	microtubule
metle	metal	microbbicide	microbicide
metoragia	metrorrhagia	microewave diathermy machine	
metradinia	metrodynia	... microwave diathermy machine	
-metree (suff)	-metry	microrganism	microorganism
metroarhajia	metrorrhagia	microsefalic	microcephalic
metrytis	metritis	microserjery	microsurgery
mett- (pre)	met-	*microssporum*	*Microsporum*
metta- (pre)	meta-	midbrane	midbrain
mettabolic acidosis		middel ear	middle ear
.... metabolic acidosis		middline	midline
mettacarpus	metacarpus	middtemporal	midtemporal
mettakromasia	metachromasia	middwife	midwife
mettamur	metamer**	midel finger	middle finger
mettapon	metopon**	midle cuneiform ...	middle cuneiform
mettastasis	metastasis**	Midline	MEDLINE
mettatarsis	metatarsus	midwifry	midwifery
-metter (suff)	-meter	mie- (pre)	mye-
mettermorfosis	metamorphosis**	-miellia (suff)	-myelia
mettopeon	metopion**	migretory	migratory
mettr- (pre)	metr-	miker- (pre)	micr-
mettri- (pre)	metri-	mikerocefalus	microcephalus**
mettropecsy	metropexy	mikro- (pre)	micro-
Mettycaine	Metycaine	mikrofilament	microfilament
metzole	metazoal**	mikrollia	microglia**
mezamorf	mesomorph	mikroscopy	microscopy
mezenterick	mesenteric	milagram	milligram
mezio- (pre)	mesio-	Milan	Mylan
mezocolon	mesocolon	mile- (pre)	myel-
mialgia	myalgia	mileo- (pre)	myelo-
miasthenia	myasthenia	mili- (pre)	milli-
miatonia	myatonia**	milignant	malignant
miatonya	myatonia**	milin sheath	myelin sheath
mic- (pre)	myc-	militis	myelitis
micertome	microtome	milk free	milk-free
michanotherepy	mechanotherapy	milkleg	milk leg
mick- (pre)	myc-	milk-let-down-reflecks	
micksture	mixture	.... milk letdown reflex	
mickterition	micturition	milk of bizmuth	milk of bismuth
mickvuh	mikvah	milk of maggnesia	
mico- (pre)	myco-	.... milk of magnesia	
micobacterium	mycobacterium	millium	milium

Incorrect	Correct	Incorrect	Correct
Milltown	**Miltown**	mixedema	**myxedema**
millyew	**milieu**	mixo- (pre)	**myxo-**
milyary	**miliary****	mixoid cist	**myxoid cyst**
Minematter disease		mmr vaccine	**MMR vaccine**
	Minamata disease	moantaje	**montage**
miner	**minor****	mobeel	**mobile**
mineralorticoid	**mineralocorticoid**	mobille	**mobile**
miner calyx	**minor calyx**	modall	**modal****
miner operation	**minor operation**	moddel	**model****
minerral water	**mineral water**	modefide radical mastectomy	
minerz asthma	**miner's asthma**		**modified radical mastectomy**
minimmal brain dysfunction		modrayt	**moderate**
	minimal brain dysfunction	moebeuss	**Möbius**
minir tranquiliser		moed	**mode**
	minor tranquilizer	moedality	**modality**
minneim	**minium****	moled	**mold****
Minner	**Minor****	moll	**mole**
minneral oil	**mineral oil**	mollasses	**molasses**
minnimumm	**minimum****	mollecular	**molecular**
minny-pill	**mini-pill**	mollecule	**molecule**
minor sergery	**minor surgery**	mollers	**molars**
minral	**mineral**	molor	**molar**
mio- (pre)	**myo-**	molte	**molt****
miocarditis	**myocarditis**	monachromait	**monochromate****
miocardium	**myocardium**	monafasea	**monophasia****
mioma	**myoma**	monagomy	**monogamy****
miopic	**myopic**	monagraf	**monograph**
miotaktic	**myotactic****	monanukleosis	**mononucleosis**
mirer-imaging	**mirror imaging**	monawral	**monaural**
miricle drug	**miracle drug**	monce pubis	**mons pubis**
miset/o- (pre)	**mycet/o-**	monefagea	**monophagia****
misetoma	**mycetoma**	mongilism	**mongolism**
-misette (suff)	**-mycette**	monikromatt	**monochromat****
-misin (suff)	**-mycin**	monileal	**monilial****
misoginee	**misogyny****	monillial vaginitis	
misoglia	**mesoglia****		**monilial vaginitis**
misscariage	**miscarriage**	*monilya*	***Monilia*****
missogany	**misogamy****	monky viris	**monkey virus**
misst	**missed**	monn- (pre)	**mon-**
mitakondria	**mitochondria**	monnacockus	**monococcus**
Mitleschmerz	**mittelschmerz**	monnamanya	**monomania**
mitril valve disease		monniter	**monitor**
	mitral valve disease	monno- (pre)	**mono-**
mittrel	**mitral**	monnocside	**monoxide**
mitturition	**mituriction**	monnogany	**monogony****
mitymicin	**mitomycin**	monnonucular phagocyte system	
mix- (pre)	**myx-**		**mononuclear phagocyte system**

Incorrect	Correct
monns veneris	**mons veneris**
monockuler	**monocular**
monoliasis	**moniliasis**
monomine oxadase inhibitors	
	monamine or
	manoamine oxidase inhibitors
monosakaride	**monosaccharide**
monosinnaptic reflex	
	monosynaptic reflex
monosite	**monocyte**
monozigottic	**monozygotic**
monthly's	**monthlies**
moocosa	**mucosa**
moocosel	**mucosal**
moodswings	**mood swings**
mootant	**mutant**
moovenent	**movement**
moran	**moron**
morbidd	**morbid**
morbiddity rate	**morbidity rate**
morchuary	**mortuary**
morebidity	**morbidity**
morebund	**moribund**
morefia	**morphea****
morening glory seeds	
	morning glory seeds
-morephic (suff)	**-morphic**
moretallity	**mortality**
morf- (pre)	**morph-**
-morf (suff)	**-morph**
-morfizm (suff)	**-morphism**
morfo- (pre)	**morpho-**
morfology	**morphology**
morg	**morgue**
morning sicness	**morning sickness**
morpheen	**morphine**
morrbific	**morbific**
morrbus	**morbus**
morrphya	**morphia****
mortefy	**mortify**
moshion sickness	**motion sickness**
moshun	**motion**
motenewron	**motoneuron**
moter end plate	**motor end plate**
moter function	**motor function**

Incorrect	Correct
moterr neuron	**motor neuron**
motillity	**motility****
motling	**mottling**
motorr nuron diseases	
	motor neuron diseases
mottor	**motor**
mourning after pill	
	morning after pill
mourning glory seeds	
	morning glory seeds
mourning sickness	
	morning sickness
mouth wash	**mouthwash**
mowth	**mouth**
moyst wart	**moist wart**
mozaic	**mosaic**
mrna	**mRNA**
mucapyurulent	**mucopurulent**
mucco- (pre)	**muco-**
mucis observation	
	mucus observation
mucopolysacharide	
	mucopolysaccharide
mucus membrane	
	mucous membrane
mucuss	**mucus****
mude	**mood**
muduller oblogata	
	medulla oblongata
mukoid	**mucoid**
mukuss	**mucous****
mulage	**moulage**
mullberry cell	**mulberry cell**
mulltiple personality	
	multiple personality
multapel	**multiple**
multaplecks	**multiplex**
multe- (pre)	**multi-**
multefaktorial inheritance	
	multifactorial inheritance
multiacksial joint	**multiaxial joint**
multipel scledrosis	
	multiple sclerosis
multiphocal murel	
	multifocal mural

Incorrect	Correct	Incorrect	Correct

multipple sklerosis ....
.... **multiple sclerosis**
mummps .... **mumps**
munchhousen syndrome ....
.... **Munchausen syndrome**
munthly period .... **monthly period**
murcery chloride ... **mercury chloride**
murcurials .... **mercurials**
Murk .... **Merck**
mus- (pre) .... **muc-**
muscel tone .... **muscle tone**
muscolaris .... **muscularis**
muscoskeletal .... **musculoskeleton**
musculer system ..... **muscular system**
muscyular atrophies ....
.... **muscular atrophies**
musi- (pre) .... **muci-**
musile relaxer .... **muscle relaxer**
musilige .... **mucilage**
musin .... **mucin**
muskle spindle .... **muscle spindle**
muskul- (pre) .... **muscul-**
muskular distrophy ....
.... **muscular dystrophy**
muskuler .... **muscular**
muskulo- (pre) .... **musculo-**
muskulous .... **musculus**
mussel fatigue .... **muscle fatigue**
mussel spazm .... **muscle spasm**
mussile-contraction headaches ....
..... **muscle-contraction headaches**
mussle .... **muscle**
mustered plaster ...... **mustard plaster**
mutalation .... **mutilation**
mutashion .... **mutation**
mutness .... **muteness**
muy- (pre) .... **my-**
myaljic encefalomyelitis ....
.... **myalgic encephalomyelitis**
myaloma .... **myeloma**
myatattic .... **myotatic****
myatonea .... **myotonia****
mycaplazms .... **mycoplasms**
mycardial infraction ....
.... **myocardial infarction**

mycrobe .... **microbe**
mycrogleal .... **microglial****
mycrosefalous .... **microcephalous****
mycrossection .... **microsection**
myecarditis .... **myocarditis**
myecology .... **mycology**
myecrosurgical free flap
technique..
.... **microsurgical free flap
technique**
myeglobin .... **myoglobin**
-myellia (suff) .... **-myelia**
mygraine .... **migraine**
mygratory .... **migratory**
myifibrils .... **myiofibrils**
myio- (pre) .... **myo-**
myistheenia gravis ....
.... **myasthenia gravis**
myjenic .... **myogenic**
mykchurate .... **micturate**
mykobakteria .... **mycobacteria**
mykrophage .... **microphage**
mykrophilaria .... **microfilaria**
mykroscopy .... **microscopy**
Myles .... **Miles**
mylin .... **myelin**
myoot .... **mute**
myoppia .... **myopia**
myoses .... **miosis****
myosin ....**myosin**
myosis .... **meiosis****
myotics ....**miotics**
-myset (suff) .... **-mycette**
-mysin (suff) .... **-mycin**
mysthenia .... **myasthenia**
mytonea .... **myotonia****
mytosis .... **mitosis**
myucin .... **mucin**
myucus plack .... **mucous plaque**
myutagen .... **mutagen**
myute .... **mute**
myutent .... **mutant**

57

N

nacc- (pre) .... **nac-**
nacco- (pre) .... **naco-**
nacent .... **nascent**
nacheral childberth ....
.... **natural childbirth**
nachur .... **nature**
nachural immunity ....
.... **natural immunity**
nad .... **NAD**
nail-fold .... **nail fold**
naip ....**nape**
nakid .... **naked**
nale .... **nail**
nale biting .... **nail-biting**
nammat- (pre) .... **nemat-**
nann- (pre) .... **nan-**
nanno- (pre) .... **nano-**
nannus .... **nanus**
napken .... **napkin**
napta ....**naphtha**
nark- (pre) .... **narc-**
narkalepsy .... **narcolepsy**
narko- (pre) .... **narco-**
narkottic .... **narcotic**
narowing .... **narrowing**
narrcotherapy .... **narcotherapy**
narsisism .... **narcissism**
narsistic .... **narcissistic**
nashonal health .... **national health**
nasil discharge .... **nasal discharge**
nasofaringeal .... **nasopharyngeal**
nasofarinx .... **nasopharynx**
nass- (pre) ....**nas-**
nassi- (pre) ....**nasi-**
nassi plikas .... **nasi plica**
nasso- (pre) ....**naso-**
nassolacrimal duct ....
.... **nasolacrimal duct**
natel .... **natal**
nateropithy .... **naturopathy**
-nathus (suff) .... **-gnathus**
nationel institute of health ....
.... **National Institutes of Health**
nativ dextran .... **native dextran**
nativvism .... **nativism**

natt- (pre) ....**nat-**
natti- (pre)...................................**nati-**
naturapathic doctor ....
.... **naturopathic doctor**
nausha gravidarum ....
.... **nausea gravidarum**
naval string .... **navel string**
nawsea .... **nausea****
nawsheated .... **nauseated**
nawzheant .... **nauseant**
naycherapathy .... **naturopathy**
naychur .... **nature**
naysal cavity .... **nasal cavity**
naysil sinus .... **nasal sinus**
naysofarynx .... **nasopharynx**
naysogastric .... **nasogastric**
naysopharyngeal .... **nasopharyngeal**
nayvel .... **navel**
naz- (pre) ....**nas-**
nazal... **nasal**
nazi- (pre) ....**nasi-**
nazo- (pre) ....**naso-**
nazolabial subaceous plugs ....
.... **nasolabial sebaceous plugs**
neanalytic psychology ....
.... **neoanalytic psychology**
neaplazm ....**neoplasm**
nears... **nares**
nebilizer .... **nebulizer**
nebothian .... **nabothian**
nebyulizer .... **nebulizer**
neckbrase .... **neck brace**
neckr- (pre) .... **necr-**
neckro- (pre) .... **necro-**
neckrofilia .... **necrophilia**
neckrotic .... **necrotic****
nee..**knee**
needel .... **needle**
neeoplasms .... **neoplasms**
neersightedness .... **nearsightedness**
neersited........................... **nearsighted**
neevus .... **nevus****
neferolithiasis .... **nephrolithiasis**
neffron unit .... **nephron unit**
-neffros (suff) .... **nephros**

nefr- (pre) .... **nephr-**
nefrectomy .... **nephrectomy**
-nefric (suff) .... **-nephric**
nefritis .... **nephritis**
nefro- (pre) .... **nephro-**
nefrology .... **nephrology**
nefrosklerosis .... **nephrosclerosis**
nefrotoxic .... **nephrotoxic**
negettive test result ....
.... **negative test result**
negitive .... **negative**
negitive feedback ....
.... **negative feedback**
neglegible .... **negligible**
nek .... **neck**
nekrafilly .... **necrophily**
nekrosis .... **necrosis**
neman .... **mnemon**
Nemettoda .... **Nematoda****
nemmato- (pre) .... **nemato-**
nemmatoed .... **nematode****
Nemmbutal .... **Nembutal**
nemonics .... **mnemonics**
-nemy (suff) .... **-nomy**
nenate .... **neonate**
neomicin .... **neomycin**
neonatle .... **neonatal**
neonetorem .... **neonatorum**
Neopronntosil .... **Neoprontosil**
nepheritis .... **nephritis**
nepherolithotomy .... **nephrolithotomy**
nephralogy .... **nephrology**
nephrytis .... **nephritis**
nerotic .... **neurotic****
nerotic depression ....
.... **neurotic depression**
nerrotomy .... **neurotomy**
nerrvo- (pre) .... **nervo-**
nerrvuss .... **nervus****
nerse .... **nurse**
nerse midwife .... **nurse-midwife**
nersery .... **nursery**
nervee .... **nervi****
nerv groath factor ....
.... **nerve growth factor**
nerviss breakdown ....
.... **nervous breakdown**
nervossa anjina .... **nervosa angina**

nervus system .... **nervous system**
nesstatherapy .... **nestotherapy**
nestytherepay .... **nestitherapy**
neucleohistone .... **nucleohistone**
neumatometer .... **pneumatometer**
neumococcal infections ....
.... **pneumococcal infections**
neumococcus microorganism ....
..... **pneumococcus microorganism**
neumocystis carinii pneumonia ....
.... *Pneumocystis carinii* **pneumonia**
neumonectomy .... **pneumonectomy**
neumonia .... **pneumonia**
neurasurgery .... **neurosurgery**
neuroraphy .... **neurorrhaphy**
neurrosis .... **neurosis**
neuterophil .... **neutrophil**
neutrafil exudation ....
.... **neutrophil exudation**
newcal .... **nucal**
newcleeye .... **nuclei**
newcleo- (pre) .... **nucleo-**
newcleus .... **nucleus**
newmanitis .... **pneumonitis**
newmatic .... **pneumatic**
newmoconiosis .... **pneumoconiosis**
newmocystis carinii pneumonia ......
.... *Pneumocystis carinii* **pneumonia**
newmogram .... **pneumogram**
newmograph .... **pneumograph**
newmonia .... **pneumonia**
newralgia .... **neuralgia**
newrel .... **neural**
newright .... **neurit** or **neurite**
newrodermitits .... **neurodermatitis**
newroesiphilid .... **neurosyphilid****
newrogenic .... **neurogenic**
newronel .... **neuronal**
newrotransmitter .... **neurotransmitter**
newtral .... **neutral**
nickoteen .... **nicotine**
nickotinamide addenine
dinucleotide ....
.... **nicotinamide adenine
dinucleotide**
nicktatation .... **nictitation**
nicktation .... **nictation**
nifralgia .... **nephralgia**

Incorrect	Correct
nightrite	**nitrite****
night sweets	**night sweats**
nigphobia	**pnigphobia**
nikthamide	**nikethamide**
nilon	**nylon**
nimf	**nymph**
nimfo- (pre)	**nympho-**
nimphomania	**nymphomania**
nioplasm	**neoplasm**
niple	**nipple**
nippa sugar	**nipa sugar**
nippel	**nipple**
niseria	*Neisseria*
nish	**niche**
nish sell	**niche cell**
nistagmus	**nystagmus**
nistatin	**nystatin**
nite blindness	**night blindness**
nitemare	**nightmare**
nitergin	**nitrogen**
niteroglicerin	**nitroglycerin**
nitragen	**nitrogen**
nitrus oxide	**nitrous oxide**
nobel gas	**noble gas**
nocht	**notch**
nock-knee	**knock-knee**
nockshus	**noxious**
nocktambulism	**noctambulism**
nockternal	**nocturnal**
nocternil	**nocturnal**
noddle	**nodule**
noddosem	**nodosum**
nodduler	**nodular**
nodle	**nodal**
nodoes	**nodose****
nodossa	**nodosa**
nody	**nodi****
noed	**node****
noeds of Ranvier	**nodes of Ranvier**
noedus	**nodus****
noll	**Knoll**
nome- (pre)	**nomo-**
nomer	**noma****
nomma	**noma****
noncontribetary	**noncontributory**
nonenvasive surgery	**noninvasive surgery**

Incorrect	Correct
nonespecific therapy	**nonspecific therapy**
nonfuncktionning	**nonfunctioning**
nonna	**nona****
nonopperible tumor	**nonoperable tumor**
nonspesific	**nonspecific**
nonspessific vaginitis	**nonspecific vaginitis**
noocleoprotein	**nucleoprotein**
nooklear medicine	**nuclear medicine**
noomocystis carinii pneumonia	*Pneumocystis carinii* **pneumonia**
noomonic plague	**pneumonic plague**
noorarn	**neuron**
noorologist	**neurologist**
nooron	**neuron**
nootrient	**nutrient**
nootrilize	**neutralize**
nopathia	**naupathia**
norjestrel	**norgestrel**
norlesstrin	**Norlestrin**
norme- (pre)	**norm-**
normeacktive	**normoactive**
normeblast	**normoblast**
normel	**normal**
normeo- (pre)	**normo-**
normly	**normally**
norpinepherine	**norepinephrine**
norrethinodrel	**norethynodrel**
nortthindrine	**norethindrone**
nosa- (pre)	**noso-**
noseeceptor	**nociceptor**
nosi- (pre)	**noci-**
noss- (pre)	**nos-**
nosso- (pre)	**noso-**
nossology	**nosology**
nosstril	**nostril**
note- (pre)	**noto-**
notefiable disease	**notifiable disease**
notefy	**notify**
notsh	**notch**
nott- (pre)	**not-**
notto- (pre)	**noto-**

Incorrect	Correct	Incorrect	Correct
novabiocin	**novobiocin**	nunnirritating diet	**nonirritating diet**
Novacain	**Novocain**	nunpalpible	**nonpalpable**
noyse	**noise**	nunsterile	**nonsterile**
noze	**nose**	Nupacaine	**Nupercaine**
nozebleed	**nosebleed**	nuphrosis	**nephrosis**
nozo- (pre)	**noso-**	nur- (pre)	**neur-**
nozocomial	**nosocomial**	nurahipafiseal	**neurohypophyseal**
Nsaids	**NSAIDs**	nuralemmal	**neurilemmal****
nuborn	**newborn**	nural tube defect	**neural tube defect**
nuborne	**newborn**	nurasifilis	**neurosyphilis****
nuckel	**knuckle**	nureology	**neurology**
nuckle- (pre)	**nucle-**	nuritis	**neuritis**
nuckleo- (pre)	**nucleo-**	nuro- (pre)	**neuro-**
nucks vomica	**nux vomica**	nurofibromatosis	**neurofibromatosis**
nucleeolus	**nucleolus**	nurohypafisial	**neurohypophysial**
nucular envelope	**nuclear envelope**	nurotic disorder	**neurotic disorder**
nuculus	**nucleus**	nurotika	**neurotica****
nueclease	**nuclease**	nurseing home	**nursing home**
nuerasthenia	**neurasthenia**	nurse middwife	**nurse-midwife**
nuerit	**neurit**	nurses' aid	**nurse's aide**
nuka	**nucha**	nurs practioner	**nurse-practitioner**
nukel chord	**nuchal cord**	nurss practishoner	
nuklear	**nuclear**		**nurse-practitioner**
nuli- (pre)	**nulli-**	nurv- (pre)	**nerv-**
nuligrevida	**nulligravida**	nurve	**nerve****
nullepara	**nullipara**	nurvi- (pre)	**nervi-****
num/o- (pre)	**pneum/o-**	nurvous	**nervous****
numatic	**pneumatic**	nuttrition	**nutrition**
numm	**numb**	nuxx vomica	**nux vomica**
numness	**numbness**	nyacin	**niacin**
numoconiosis	**pneumoconiosis**	-nyoa (suff)	**-noia**
numogastric nerve		nyocortex	**neocortex**
	pneumogastric nerve	nytrate	**nitrate****
numonia	**pneumonia**	nyt vision	**night vision**
numular	**nummular**	nyucleotidase	**nucleotidase**
nun- (pre)	**non-**	nyuralgia	**neuralgia**
nunadicting	**nonaddicting**	nyurilemma	**neurilemma****
nun compass mentiss		nyuro- (pre)	**neuro-**
	non compos mentis	nyurology	**neurology**
nunifective state		nyurotic-depressive reaction	
	noninfective state		**neurotic-depressive reaction**

O

Incorrect	Correct	Incorrect	Correct
ob	**OB**	obblitterans	**obliterans**
obbliteration	**obliteration**	obbsession	**obsession**

Incorrect	Correct	Incorrect	Correct
obbstetrical	obstetrical	oderus	odorous
obbstetrics	obstetrics	-odinia (suff)	-odynia
obbstipation	obstipation	odonntytis	odontitis
obbstruction	obstruction	-odonshia (suff)	-odontia
obcellete	obsolete	-oedont (suff)	-odont
obdurater	obturator	oeosperm	oosperm
obece	obese	offiss	office
obeecity	obesity	oforectomy	oophorectomy
obeesity	obesity	ofthalm- (pre)	ophthalm-
obgective signs	objective signs	ofthalmo- (pre)	ophthalmo-
ob-gine	OB GYN	ofthalmologist	ophthalmologist
obleak	oblique	oh- (pre)	o-
obleek	oblique	ohd	od**
obleekus	obliquus	ohrbitail	orbitale**
obsesive personality	obsessive personality	ohrganic disorder	organic disorder
obsesseve-commpulsive sychoneurosis	obsessive-compulsive psychoneurosis	ohs	os
		ohtic	otic
obsessivcompulsiv reaction	obsessive-compulsive reaction	ointmints	ointment
obtuce	obtuse	oklusion	occlusion
occippital lobe	occipital lobe	oks- (pre)	ox-
occul/o- (pre)	ocul/o-	oksidative slow fibers	oxidative slow fibers
ockipital	occipital	okso- (pre)	oxo-
ocklusive	occlusive	oktane	octane**
ockside	oxide	olefactory lobe	olfactory lobe
ockuler	ocular	-olle (suff)	-ole
ockuli	oculi	ollegojenic	oligogenic**
ockult blood	occult blood	ollfactory nerve	olfactory nerve
oclusal	occlusal	ollfactry	olfactory
oclution	occlusion	olliagenous	oleaginous
octain	octane**	ollig- (pre)	olig-
octin	octan**	olligo- (pre)	oligo-
oculamotor nerve	oculomotor nerve	olligoegenix	oligogenics**
ocupit	occiput	olligofrenia	oligophrenia
ocurring sporadicly	occurring sporadically	ollive oil	olive oil
		omeega	omega
ocyte	oocyte	omfal- (pre)	omphal-
ocyupational therapy	occupational therapy	omfalo- (pre)	omphalo-
		-omma (suff)	-oma
odde	odd**	ommbudsman	ombudsman
oddont- (pre)	odont-	ommentim	omentum
oddonto- (pre)	odonto-	-onckia (suff)	-onchia
odentoma	odontoma	onich- (pre)	onych-
oder	odor	-onichia (suff)	-onychia
		onicho- (pre)	onycho-
		onixis	onyxis
		onko- (pre)	oncho-
		onnanizm	onanism

Incorrect	Correct	Incorrect	Correct
onn-call	**on-call**	opration	**operation**
onnch- (pre)	**onch-**	optamal lenth	**optimal length**
onncho- (pre)	**oncho-**	opthalmascope	**ophthalmoscope**
onncology	**oncology****	optick kiasma	**optic chiasma**
-onnichium (suff)	**-onychium**	optik nerve	**optic nerve**
onnykosis	**onychosis**	optishan	**optician**
on-set	**onset**	opto- (pre)	**opto-**
ontojiny	**ontogeny**	optommetrist	**optometrist**
oofor- (pre)	**oophor-**	opyum	**opium**
ooforo- (pre)	**oophoro-**	orafis	**orifice**
oogimy	**oogamy**	orall	**oral****
ooh- (pre)	**oo-**	orall contraceptive	
oojenesis	**oogenesis**		**oral contraceptive**
opake	**opaque**	oralle	**orale****
opasification	**opacification**	orbatal cavity	**orbital cavity**
opasity	**opacity**	orbickularis	**orbicularis**
opeate	**opiate**	orbickuler	**orbicular**
operrative risk	**operative risk**	orchitomee	**orchotomy****
operrtunist	**opportunist**	ordelly	**orderly**
opeum	**opium**	-orecksia (suff)	**-orexia**
opfalmoplegia	**ophthalmoplegia**	oreental	**oriental**
-ophthallmia (suff)	**-ophthalmia**	oreganic brane syndrome	
ophthallmic nerve			**organic brain syndrome**
	ophthalmic nerve	oregin	**origin**
ophthomology	**ophthalmology**	orel polio vaccine	
opin-heart surgery			**oral polio vaccine**
	open-heart surgery	orethotoppic	**orthotopic****
oponent	**opponent**	orfan	**orphan**
oposing marjins	**opposing margins**	orfice	**orifice**
opperating room	**operating room**	organ therapy	**organotherapy**
opperent	**operant**	organnels	**organelles**
opperible canser	**operable cancer**	organnic	**organic**
opperitive	**operative**	organn of Corti	**organ of Corti**
-oppia (suff)	**-opia**	orgasstic disfunction	
oppisth- (pre)	**opisth-**		**orgastic dysfunction**
oppistho- (pre)	**opistho-**	orgazm	**orgasm**
oppsia (suff)	**-opsia**	orgenism	**organism**
oppsinins	**opsonins**	orgen sistem	**organ system**
oppsonic therapy	**opsonic therapy**	orgin	**organ**
oppt- (pre)	**opt-**	orgin transplant	**organ transplant**
oppthalm- (pre)	**ophthalm-**	orho- (pre)	**orrho-**
oppthalmia	**ophthalmia**	oril sergin	**oral surgeon**
oppthalmo- (pre)	**ophthalmo-**	oril surgery	**oral surgery**
opptic	**optic**	orisenin	**oryzenin**
opptical	**optical**	orki- (pre)	**orchi-**
opptick- (pre)	**optic-**	-orkidism (suff)	**-orchidism**
oppticko- (pre)	**optico-**	orkio- (pre)	**orchio-**
opptometry	**optometry**	-orkism (suff)	**-orchism**

Incorrect	Correct	Incorrect	Correct
orkitis	orchitis	ostealogy	osteology**
orofaringeal	oropharyngeal	osteapath	osteopath
orr- (pre)	or-	osteopporosis	osteoporosis
orra	ora**	ostilojia	osteologia**
orral cavity	oral cavity	ostioarthritis	osteoarthritis
orrbit	orbit	ostiochondr- (pre)	osteochondr-
-orrexia (suff)	-orexia	ostiochondro- (pre)	osteochondro-
orrgan/o- (pre)	organ/o-	ostiopathy	osteopathy
orrigen	origin	ostoblast	osteoblast
orriginal	original	ostrus	estrus**
orris	oris	osty- (pre)	oste-
orrkid/o- (pre)	orchid/o-	ostya	ostia**
orro- (pre)	oro-	ostyo- (pre)	osteo-
orropharyngeal	oropharyngeal	ostyoclasis	osteoclasis
orrth- (pre)	orth-	otalaringology	otolaryngology
orrtho- (pre)	ortho-	otescope	otoscope
orthadiagraph	orthodiagraph	otimycosis	otomycosis
orthatropick	orthotropic**	otittis	otitis
orthepedik surgeon		otoesklerosis	otosclerosis
	orthopedic surgeon	otollogy	otology
orthestetic	orthostatic	otorinolarynjology	
orthidontics	orthodontics		otorhinolaryngology
orthoedontist	orthodontist	ott- (pre)	ot-
orthopeedics	orthopedics	ottalgia	otalgia
osafication	ossification	-ottic (suff)	-otic
ose- (pre)	osse-	otto- (pre)	oto-
oseo- (pre)	osseo-	ottorhea	otorrhea
oseomucoid	osseomucoid	-ouss (suff)	-ous
oseous	osseous	outbrake	outbreak
osetectomy	ostectomy	out pashent	outpatient
osiculer chane	ossicular chain	out-put	output
osificans	ossificans	ova-active	overactive
-osizes (suff)	-osises	ovabite	overbite
osmotick	osmotic	ovaburdened heart	
osmottic pressure	osmotic pressure		overburdened heart
osoan	ozone	ovadose	overdose
-osses (suff)	-oses	ovaduct	oviduct
ossilagraf	oscillograph	ovail	oval**
-ossis (suff)	-osis	ovarries	ovaries
ossmoreceptor	osmoreceptor	ovaryan	ovarian
ossteal	ostial**	ovee- (pre)	ovi-
ossteitis	osteitis	oveeo- (pre)	ovio-
ossteo- (pre)	osteo-	ovel	oval**
ossteoclast	osteoclast	ovelbumin	ovalbumin
-ossteoma (suff)	-osteoma	overberdened heart	
ossteomilitis	osteomyelitis		overburdened heart
-ossteon (suff)	-osteon	overcedation	oversedation
ossteotomy	osteotomy	overdoce	overdose

Incorrect	Correct
over-flow	overflow
overian follicle	ovarian follicle
overkompensation	overcompensation
over-lay	overlay
overperscribe	overprescribe
overrt	overt
over-wait	overweight
oviglobelan	ovoglobulin
ovim	ovum
ovotesstis	ovotestis
ovovittelin	ovovitellin
ovry	ovary
ovval window	oval window
ovvar- (pre)	ovar-
ovvaro- (pre)	ovaro-
ownce	ounce
owtcroping	outcropping
owter ear	outer ear
owtflow track	outflow tract
oxaddative fast fibers	oxidative fast fibers
oxasepamm	oxazepam
oxedative fosforylation	oxidative phosphorylation
oxeehemoglobin	oxyhemoglobin

Incorrect	Correct
oxegen	oxygen
oxejjen therapy	oxygen therapy
oxicillin	oxacillin
oxigen mask	oxygen mask
oxijen tent	oxygen tent
oxintic cells	oxyntic cells
oxitocic	oxytocic
oxx- (pre)	ox-
oxxidative	oxidative
oxxo- (pre)	oxo-
oxxygen tank	oxygen tank
oxyjenator	oxygenator
oxytettrasycline	oxytetracycline
oxytokin	oxytocin
-oyd (suff)	-oid
oyl glasnd	oil gland
oyntment	ointment
-oze (suff)	-ose
ozm- (pre)	osm-
-ozmia (suff)	-osmia
ozmics	osmics
ozmo- (pre)	osmo-
ozmolarity	osmolarity
ozmosis	osmosis
ozmotic shock	osmotic shock

P

Incorrect	Correct
pac	pack
pacive smoking	passive smoking
packt	packed
Padock	Paddock
-page (suff)	-pague
-pagge (suff)	-pague
pail- (pre)	pale-
pailo- (pre)	paleo-
painkiler	painkiller
pairesis	paresis**
pair revue organization	peer review organization
pairz	pairs
Pakinsonz disease	Parkinson's disease

Incorrect	Correct
palade	pelade
palatoe- (pre)	palato-
palbible	palpable
paleative treatment	palliative treatment
paletine	palatine
pallatine tonsil	palatine tonsil
pallato- (pre)	palato-
paller	pallor
pallete	palate
palleum	pallium
pallpate	palpate**
pallpation	palpation**
pallzy	palsy
palpatait	palpitate**

Incorrect	Correct	Incorrect	Correct
palpetation	**palpitation****	parafilia	**paraphilia**
palpitary percussion		paragoric	**paregoric**
	palpatory percussion	-parah (suff)	**-para**
palprabrel	**palpebral**	paralisis	**paralysis**
palyiative	**palliative**	paralldehide	**paraldehyde**
palzy	**palsy**	parameddic	**paramedic**
pamar	**palmar**	parannoya	**paranoia**
pam sugar	**palm sugar**	parapereesis	**paraparesis**
panckreatic amilase		parapleejia	**paraplegia**
	pancreatic amylase	parapleksia	**paraplexia**
pancrease	**pancreas**	parasychology	**parapsychology**
pancreesimin	**pancreozymin**	parasyttic	**paracytic****
pancreetitis	**pancreatitis**	parathiroyd	**parathyroid**
pane	**pain**	paratifoid fever	**paratyphoid fever**
paneful	**painful**	parchurition	**parturition**
paneless	**painless**	paredocks	**paradox**
panesea	**panacea**	pareesis	**paresis****
panick	**panic**	parekimel	**parachymal**
pankreet- (pre)	**pancreat-**	pare-shaped heart	
pankreeto- (pre)	**pancreato-**		**pear-shaped heart**
pann- (pre)	**pan-**	paridoxical sleep	**paradoxical sleep**
panncreatic juice	**pancreatic juice**	parinoid skizophrenia	
panndemic	**pandemic****		**paranoid schizophrenia**
pannel	**panel**	-paris (suff)	**-parous**
pannis	**pannus****	parisight	**parasite****
pannous	**panus****	parisitic	**paracytic****
pannt	**pant**	parissitic	**parasitic****
panntaphobea	**pantaphobia****	parithyroid gland	
pantefobia	**pantophobia****		**parathyroid gland**
papal/o- (pre)	**papill/o-**	Park-Davis	**Parke-Davis**
papane	**papain**	parkinnsonism	**parkinsonism**
papelossa	**papulosa**	Parkinsonz disease	
papeus	**pappus****		**Parkinson's disease**
papila	**papilla****	parnoid personality	
paploma virus	**papilloma virus**		**paranoid personality**
papose	**pappose****	parocksismal	**paroxysmal**
Pappanicolaou test		paroksizm	**paroxysm**
	Papanicolaou test	parr- (pre)	**par-**
pappavarine	**papaverine**	parra	**para**
pappillary	**papillary**	parracasin	**paracasein**
pappiniform plexus		parrafin	**paraffin**
	papiniform plexus	parraglosa	**paraglossa****
papp smear	**Pap smear**	parrahormone	**parahormone**
Papp test	**Pap test**	parralitic	**paralytic**
pappula	**papula****	parrallax	**parallax**
papyule	**papule****	parrallel	**parallel**
paracytology	**parasitology**	parrameter	**parameter****
paradocks	**paradox**	parranasel	**paranasal**

Incorrect	Correct	Incorrect	Correct
parrasimpathetic	**parasympathetic**	pathejenic	**pathogenic**
parrasitic	**parasitic****	pathelogic	**pathologic**
parrekeratosis	**parakeratosis**	pathelogist	**pathologist**
parrenchimatous	**parenchymatous**	pathenejenesis	**parthenogenesis**
parreneral	**parenteral**	patheo- (pre)	**patho-**
parrent	**parent**	pathijens	**pathogens**
parrer- (pre)	**para-**	-pathik (suff)	**-pathic**
parrethiroid hormone		pathmimmicry	**pathomimicry**
	parathyroid hormone	pathoe- (pre)	**patho-**
parrglossia	**paraglossia****	pathollogy	**pathology**
parrietal cells	**parietal cells**	pathwhey	**pathway**
parrinchima	**parenchyma**	-pathya (suff)	**-pathia**
parro- (pre)	**paro-**	patint	**patent****
parrotid	**parotid**	patint advocacy	**patient advocacy**
parrotid gland	**parotid gland**	patition	**partition**
parrs	**pars**	patsh	**patch**
parrshally	**partially**	patsh test	**patch test**
parrts	**parts****	pattella	**patella****
parshall	**partial**	pattent medicine	**patent medicine**
parsyesis	**paracyesis****	paturnitty	**paternity**
parties	**partes****	Pavlove	**Pavlov**
paruthirin	**parathyrin**	pawnch	**paunch****
paryetal lobe	**parietal lobe**	payne	**pain**
parytal	**parietal**	paytency	**patency**
pasciv-aggresive reaction		Pazet's disease	**Paget's disease**
	passive-aggressive reaction	pea	**pia****
pascive smoking	**passive smoking**	pealing of skin	**peeling of skin**
paseje	**passage**	peccten	**pecten****
pasemaker	**pacemaker**	pecctus	**pectus****
pashent	**patient****	pecktin	**pectin****
pasive-agressive personality		pecktis	**pectus**
	passive-aggressive personality	pecktoris	**pectoris**
pasive-dependants reaction		pecteral fashia	**pectoral fascia**
	passive-dependence reaction	pectrall gerdle	**pectoral girdle**
passif immunity	**passive immunity**	pedaculosis	**pediculosis**
passinian corpussle		pedafilia	**pedophilia**
	pacinian corpuscle	peddicule	**pedicule**
pasturella	***Pasteurella***	peddicullous	**pediculous****
patassium	**potassium**	peddiculosis	**pediculosis**
patel/o- (pre)	**patell/o-**	peddle	**pedal**
pateler	**patellar****	peddodontics	**pedodontics**
paten	**patten****	pedikulos	**pediculus****
patensy	**patency**	pedikulosis public	
patern	**pattern****		**pediculosis pubic**
pathagen	**pathogen**	pedoncle	**peduncule**
pathe- (pre)	**path-**	Pee and Vee	**P and V**
-pathe (suff)	**-path**	peed- (pre)	**ped-**
-pathee (suff)	**-pathy**	peedeatric	**pediatric**

Incorrect	Correct	Incorrect	Correct
peedio- (pre)	pedio-	percordial	precordial
peediatrics	pediatrics	percushon	percussion
peedo- (pre)	pedo-	percuteanus	percutaneous
pee-wave	P wave	perdissposing cause	
pegg	peg		predisposing cause
pektoral	pectoral	perdominent	predominant
pektous	pectous**	Perdue Frederick	
pelagra	pellagra		Purdue Frederick
-pelic (suff)	-pellic	pere- (pre)	per-
pelikulla	pellicula**	pereadontal disease	
pellada	pelada		periodontal disease
pelleculer	pellicular**	perecardial disease	
pellution	pollution		pericardial disease
pellv- (pre)	pelv-	peredontics	periodontics
pellvi- (pre)	pelvi-	pereenatology	perinatology
pellvic	pelvic	perenneal	perineal**
pellvic girdle	pelvic girdle	pereosteum	periosteum
pelvik inflamatory disease		perestalsis	peristalsis
	pelvic inflammatory disease	perfenazine	perphenazine
pelvus	pelvis**	perferated	perforated
pemfigis	pemphigus	perferation	perforation
pendalus	pendulous	pergative	purgative
-penea (suff)	-penia	pergressive	progressive
penecillin	penicillin	peridontics	periodontics
penel	penile	periferal resistance	
penetrants	penetrance		peripheral resistance
penil prosthesis	penile prosthesis	periferel	peripheral
penn- (pre)	pen-	perikarditis	pericarditis
penno- (pre)	peno-	peristatic waves	peristaltic waves
penntosan	pentosan	perliminary	preliminary
penntose sugar	pentose sugar	permenant	permanent
pentabarbital	pentobarbital	permisiveness	permissiveness
pentithal	Pentothal	peroneel nerve	peroneal nerve
penus	penis	peroneum	perineum
peppsin	pepsin	perossis	pyrosis
pepptide	peptide	peroxxisome	peroxisome
pepptones	peptones	perpera	purpura
-pepsya (suff)	-pepsia	perpura	purpura
Pepta-Bizmol	Pepto-Bismol	perr	per**
peptadase	peptidase	perramidal newron	
peptick ulser	peptic ulcer		pyramidal neuron
peptoan	peptone	perrcussion hammer	
perasite	pericyte**		percussion hammer
peraton- (pre)	periton-	perrenatal	perinatal**
peratono- (pre)	peritono-	perrenial	perennial
percistant	persistent	perrianal	perianal

perriaortic .... **periaortic**

perricardial cavity ....

.... **pericardial cavity**

perriodic .... **periodic**

perriodontist .... **periodontist**

perriostium .... **periosteum**

perristalsis .... **peristalsis**

perristeal .... **periosteal**

perritic rash .... **pruritic rash**

perritonitis .... **peritonitis**

perronial .... **peroneal****

perroxide .... **peroxide**

perrsonal health care ....

.... **personal health care**

perrsonalty theory ....

.... **personality theory**

perrycardium .... **pericardium**

perrytoneal .... **peritoneal****

persacution complex ....

.... **persecution complex**

perscribed .... **prescribed**

persennality disorder ....

.... **personality disorder**

perseption .... **perception**

personnal indifference ....

.... **personal indifference**

persperation .... **perspiration**

persumptive .... **presumptive**

pervurt .... **pervert**

pery- (pre) .... **peri-**

peryod .... **period**

peryodontal membrane ....

.... **periodontal membrane**

pess .... **pes****

pessry .... **pessary**

pesstilence .... **pestilence**

pestaside .... **pesticide**

petralatum .... **petrolatum**

petroezal .... **petrosal****

petrolleum jelly .... **petroleum jelly**

pet-scan .... **PET scan**

pettrossa .... **petrosa****

petty mal .... **petit mal**

pewbovaginal muscle ....

.... **pubovaginal muscle**

pewpillary .... **pupillary**

pewtrid bronkitis ... **putrid bronchitis**

-pexxy (suff) .... **-pexy**

phagacyte .... **phagocyte**

phagoecitosis .... **phagocytosis**

-phaige (suff) .... **-phage**

phallanges .... **phalanges**

pharinjopalatine arch ....

.... **pharyngopalatine arch**

pharmak/o- (pre) .... **pharmac/o-**

pharmecutical .... **pharmaceutical**

pharmekotherapy ....

.... **pharmacotherapy**

pharmicologist .... **pharmacologist**

pharmicy .... **pharmacy**

pharmocopea .... **pharmacopoeia**

phaylanx .... **phalanx**

phazic .... **phasic**

phazo- (pre) .... **phaso-**

pheakromocytoma ....

.... **pheochromocytoma**

pheenobarbital .... **phenobarbital**

pheenol .... **phenol**

pheenotype .... **phenotype**

phenathisillin .... **phenethicillin**

phenellalinine .... **phenylalanine**

phenezine .... **phenelzine**

phennazone .... **phanazone**

phennomenelogical approach ....

.... **phenomenological approach**

phenoles .... **phenols**

phenolfthalin .... **phenolphthalein**

phensiclidine .... **phencyclidine**

pheronome .... **pheromone**

philim .... **phylum****

-phill .... **-phil**

philojeny .... **phylogeny**

phimossis .... **phimosis**

phiseek .... **physique****

phiseology .... **physiology**

phisi- (pre) .... **physi-**

phisical .... **physical**

phisio- (pre) .... **physio-**

phisiologic .... **physiologic**

phisyatrisst .... **physiatrist****

phisycian .... **physician**

phit- (pre) .... **phyt-**

phito- (pre) ....phyto-
phlebbotimy ....phlebotomy
-phobea (suff) ....-phobia
-phobick (suff) ....-phobic
phonacardiogram ....
.........................phonocardiogram
phonagramm ....phonogram
phonecardeography.........................
.....................phonocardiography
-phoney (suff) ....-phony
-phorea (suff) ....-phoria
phosferus.....................phosphorus
phosfoaminolipide ....
.....................phosphoaminolipide
phosfolipid.....................phospholipid
phosforilation ....phosphorylation
phossfean ....phosphine**
phossphoproteen ....phosphoprotein
photageen......................photogene**
photatherapy ....phototherapy
photoeplethismograph ....
...................photoplethysmograph
phrinia- (pre) ....phrenia-
phulang- (pre) ....phalang-
phulango- (pre) ....phalango-
physcal therapist ... physical therapist
physitherapist ....physiotherapist
picertoxin ....picrotoxin
pidgeon toes ....pigeon toes
pie- (pre) ....py-
pielography ....pyelography
pieloric ....pyloric
pielorus ....pylorus
pierea ....pyorrhea
pieriform ....piriform or pyriform
pierogenic ....pyrogenic**
piggmant ....pigment
pigmentossa ....pigmentosa
pigmintation ....pigmentation
pigmintry ....pigmentory
pika ....pica
pil.....................pill
pilar.....................pillar
pill- (pre) ....pil-
pilli- (pre) ....pili-
pilliated ....piliated
pillo- (pre) ....pilo-
pillomotor ....pilomotor

pilloroplasty ....pyloroplasty
pillose ....pilose**
pillowerection ....piloerection
pillus ....pilus**
pilogram ....pyelogram
pilonephritis ....pyleonephritis
pilonidal ....pilonidal
piloric ....pyloric
pimpel ....pimple
pina ....pinna
pink-diseese ....pink disease
pink eye ....pinkeye
pinneal body ....pineal body
pin-pong infection ....
.....................ping-pong infection
pio- (pre).....................pyo-
piocyanas ....pyocyanas
piocyanin ....pyocyanin
piogenic ....pyogenic**
piorrhea ....pyorrhea
piprocaine ....piperocaine
piramid.....................pyramid
pirettic ....pyretic**
pirexia ....pyrexia*
pirogenic ....pyrogenic
pirriform ....piriform or pyriform
pirrole ....pyrrole
pissiform ....pisiform
pisstin ....piston
pitersin ....pitressin
pitiriasis ....pityriasis
pittuetary gland ....pituitary gland
pitutery.....................pituitary
pivet joynt........................pivot joint
placintation ....placentation
plack ....plaque
plage ....plague
plain wart ....plane wart
plaite ....plate
plaitlet ....platelet
Planed Parinthood Federation ....
.... Planned Parenthood Federation
plane gut ....plain gut
plannta ....planta**
planntar wart.................plantar wart
planter ....plantar**
planter flechsors .... plantar flexors
plasama fractions.... plasma fractions

Incorrect	Correct	Incorrect	Correct

plaseebo .... **placebo**
plasement .... **placement**
plasenta .... **placenta**
plasentay brute .... **placentae bruit**
plasmar membrane ....
.... **plasma membrane**
plasmer cell .... **plasma cell**
plassenta .... **placenta**
plassmin .... **plasmin**
plasster .... **plaster**
plasstic surgery .... **plastic surgery**
plastidd .... **plastid**
plaszma ....**plasma****
plateopic .... **platyopic**
platlet .... **platelet**
plattlet .... **platelet**
playte .... **plate**
-plazm (suff) .... **-plasm****
plazma extender ..... **plasma extender**
plazma transfusion ....
.... **plasma transfusion**
plazmid .... **plasmid**
Plazmodeum malaria ....
.... ***Plasmodium malariae***
plazning .... **planning**
plecksuses .... **plexuses**
-pleggia (suff) .... **-plegia**
plesser .... **plessor**
pleuril cavity .... **pleural cavity**
plexxis...................... **plexus**
plexxor....................... **plexor**
plicka ....**plica**
plooral...................... **plural****
pluerisy .... **pleurisy**
plummism .... **plumbism**
plur- (pre) .... **pleur-**
plura...................... **pleura**
pluro- (pre) .... **pleuro-**
pnemonia .... **pneumonia**
pneumacistis cariny pneumonia .....
....*Pneumocystis carinii* pneumonia
pneuropathy .... **neuropathy**
pnewmothorax .... **pneumothorax**
pnoococcal infections ....
.... **pneumococcal infections**
pnumatograph .... **pneumatograph**
poc ....**pock**
pocced................. **pocked****

pocked mark .... **pockmark**
pockit .... **pocket****
poddagra ....**podagra**
podietry................... **podiatry**
podofillin .... **podophyllin**
poisinous................... **poisonous**
poisinus................... **poisonous**
poizning................... **poisoning**
poks...................... **pocks****
Polack .... **Pollack**
Polak .... **Pollak**
poleunsaturated fat ....
.... **polyunsaturated fat**
polichromatic .... **polychromatic**
policistic .... **polycystic**
polidipsia .... **polydipsia**
poliethylene .... **polyethylene**
polimixin................... **polymyxin**
polineuritis .... **polyneuritis**
polioe vaccine.............. **polio vaccine**
poliomelitis .... **poliomyelitis**
polippus .... **polypous****
pollarizing .... **polarizing**
poller...................... **polar**
polles...................... **poles****
pollimorfonucular granulocytes ......
.... **polymorphonuclear granulocytes**
pollip...................... **polyp**
pollipectomy .... **polypectomy**
pollipoid................... **polypoid**
pollishing .... **polishing**
pollus ....**polus****
polly- (pre) .... **poly-**
pollymorephous perverts ....
.... **polymorphous perverse**
pollymorf .... **polymorph**
pollypeptide ....**polypeptide**
pollypoid................... **polypoid**
pollypus .... **polypus****
poltice .... **poultice**
poluria .... **polyuria**
polynoocleotidase ... **polynucleotidase**
polynuritis .... **polyneuritis**
polyo .... **polio**
polysakridea............. **polysaccharidea**
polysistic .... **polycystic**
ponse .... **pons**

71

Incorrect	Correct
pontin	**pontine**
poolmonary ventilation	
	pulmonary ventilation
poorine bases	**purine bases**
popers	**poppers**
poplishal nerve	**popliteal nerve**
poppliteal	**popliteal**
popullar	**papular****
poreous	**porous****
porfyria	**porphyria**
porr	**pore****
porrus	**porus****
portel system	**portal system**
posative test result	
	positive test result
poschural back problem	
	postural back problem
poschure sence	**posture sense**
posible diagnosis	**possible diagnosis**
posishun	**position**
positif boan skan	
	positive bone scan
posittron emission tomograph	
	positron emission tomograph
pospartem	**postpartum**
posprandial	**postprandial**
possterior lobe disorders	
	posterior lobe disorders
possteryur	**posterior**
poste- (pre)	**post-**
postireor chamber	
	posterior chamber
postmortum	**postmortem**
postnazal drip	**postnasal drip**
postopp	**post-op**
postopperative	**postoperative**
postparttem depression	
	postpartum depression
postraumatic stress syndrome	
	posttraumatic stress syndrome
postsenatic neuron	
	postsynaptic neuron
postsergical	**postsurgical**
post term birth	**post-term birth**
post traumatic	**posttraumatic**
postumus	**posthumous**

Incorrect	Correct
potenchiation	**potentiation**
pottasium permanganate	
	potassium permanganate
pottent	**potent**
pottential	**potential**
pourr	**pour****
powch	**pouch**
poxx	**pox****
poynt	**point**
poysenous	**poisonous**
poysin	**poison****
poyson ivy	**poison ivy**
poyzon sumac	**poison sumac**
pozitive feedback	
	positive feedback
pracktitioner	**practitioner**
practise	**practice**
praktical nurse	**practical nurse**
praycocks	**praecox**
precanserus	**precancerous**
precardel vane	**precardial vein**
precawsion	**precaution**
pre-cenile	**presenile**
precenile dementia	
	presenile dementia
preddnesone	**prednisone**
predissposition	**predisposition**
pree- (pre)	**pre-**
pree-AIDES	**pre-AIDS**
pre-ecklamzia	**preeclampsia**
preemature	**premature**
preemenstral syndrome	
	premenstrual syndrome
preenatal	**prenatal****
preepuse	**prepuce**
preeterm	**preterm**
preeventiv medicine	
	preventive medicine
preevius	**previous****
preffered-provider organization	
	preferred provider organization
pregnency test	**pregnancy test**
pregnent	**pregnant**
prekanserous	**precancerous**
prekoshous puberty	
	precocious puberty

premachurely .... **prematurely**
premichure birth ...... **premature birth**
premoelar .... **premolar**
preon .... **prion**
preopperetive .... **preoperative**
preperation .... **preparation**
prepp .... **prep**
prept .... **prepped**
presaycral .... **presacral**
presher point technique ....
.... **pressure point technique**
preshure .... **pressure****
presinaptic nuron ....
.... **presynaptic neuron**
presisstolic mermer ....
.... **presystolic murmur**
presor .... **pressor****
presscription .... **prescription**
prevelance .... **prevalence**
prevenntive .... **preventive**
prevension .... **prevention**
prexisting-condition ....
.... **preexisting condition**
prezbiopia .... **presbyopia**
prezentation .... **presentation**
pricly heat .... **prickly heat**
priemary care network ....
.... **primary care network**
prievate practice ...... **private practice**
primative .... **primitive**
primery care .... **primary care**
primry .... **primary**
princcipel .... **principle****
prinsipal .... **principal****
pripism .... **priapism**
privatte insurance ....
.... **private insurance**
privit duty nurse ....
.... **private duty nurse**
prizim .... **prism**
probbing of wund ... **probing of wound**
problim .... **problem**
procaryout .... **prokaryote**
procksimal .... **proximal**
procktalgia fugacks ....
.... **proctalgia fugax**

procktology .... **proctology**
proctascope .... **proctoscope**
prodduct line extension ....
.... **product line extension**
proe- (pre)................................ **pro-**
proeb .... **probe**
proeband .... **proband**
proesesus .... **processus**
proeteous .... **proteus****
profase .... **prophase**
proffesional carer ....
.... **professional career**
proffusion .... **perfusion****
profilactic .... **prophylactic**
profoose .... **profuse**
profution .... **profusion****
progection .... **projection**
progesstin .... **progestin**
proggnosis .... **prognosis**
programed .... **programmed**
progresion .... **progression**
prohorrmone .... **prohormone**
projesterone .... **progesterone**
prokaine .... **procaine**
proklorprazine .... **prochlorperazine**
prokrasstination .... **procrastination**
prokt- (pre) .... **proct-**
prokto- (pre) .... **procto-**
prolaktin .... **prolactin**
prolaps .... **prolapse**
proleen .... **proline**
prolifferation .... **proliferation**
prollamine .... **prolamin**
prolonged layber ...... **prolonged labor**
promizine .... **promazine**
promminant anthelicks ....
.... **prominent anthelix**
proneucleus .... **pronucleus**
Pronntosil .... **Prontosil**
proon juice sputum ....
.... **prune juice sputum**
prooritus anni .... **pruritus ani**
propeen .... **propene****
prophallaxis .... **prophylaxis**
proppain .... **propane****
proppptosis .... **proptosis**

Incorrect	Correct	Incorrect	Correct
proproception	**proprioception**	prustration	**prostration**
prosedyure capture		pryor	**prior**
	procedure capture	pryvat hospital	**private hospital**
proseedure	**procedure**	psichee	**psyche**
prosess	**process**	psichic	**psychic****
prosesses	**processes**	psichoactive	**psychoactive**
prosspective payment		psichodelic	
	prospective payment		**psychedelic** or **psychodelic**
prosstate	**prostate****	psichodrama	**psychodrama**
prossthodontist	**prosthodontist**	psichotherepy	**psychotherapy**
prosstrait	**prostrate****	psighkoneurotic disorder	
prosstratic cancer	**prostatic cancer**		**psychoneurotic disorder**
prostait gland	**prostate gland**	psik- (pre)	**psych-**
prosteesis	**prosthesis**	psiko- (pre)	**psycho-**
prostitis	**prostatitis**	psikobabble	**psychobabble**
prostodontics	**prosthodontics**	psilium	**psyllium****
prostoglandin	**prostaglandin**	*psudomonas*	*Pseudomonas*
protacall	**protocol**	psychababble	**psychobabble**
protazoal diseases		psychalojical dependency	
	protozoal diseases		**psychological dependency**
prote- (pre)	**prot-**	psychasthenic reaction	
proteen	**protein****		**psychoasthenic reaction**
proteese	**protease**	psychatroppics	**psychotropics**
proteine supplement		psychepathology	**psychopathology**
	protein supplement	psychoesommatic	**psychosomatic**
proteo- (pre)	**proto-**	psychofisics	**psychophysics**
proteplazm	**protoplasm**	psychosexxual disorder	
protherombin	**prothrombin**		**psychosexual disorder**
pro-time	**protime**	psyechosomatic illness	
protimine	**protamine**		**psychosomatic illness**
protine	**protean****	psykasthenia	**psychasthenia**
protine therapy	**protein therapy**	psykomotor	**psychomotor**
protinnase	**proteinase**	psykoserjury	**psychosurgery**
protiolipide		psylocibin	**psilocybin**
	proteolipid or **proteolipide**	pterionn	**pterion****
protiose	**proteose****	pubacocksyjeus	**pubococcygeus**
protooberence	**protuberance**	pubblic health	**public health**
protosole	**protozoal****	pubik simfisis	**pubic symphysis**
protrution	**protrusion**	public helth nerse	
prottoxide of nitrogin			**Public Health Nurse**
	protoxide of nitrogen	Publick Helth Service	
protus	**proteus****		**Public Health Service**
protyolitic	**proteolytic**	public lice	**pubic lice**
provvider	**provider**	puboccocigeal muscle	
prown	**prone**		**pubococcygeal muscle**
prurytus	**pruritus**	puddendal block	**pudendal block**
prusack	**Prussack****	pul	**pull**
prusick	**prussic****	pulce	**pulse**

Incorrect	Correct	Incorrect	Correct
pullm- (pre)	**pulm-**	purrnicious anemia	
pullmo- (pre)	**pulmo-**		**pernicious anemia**
pullmonary	**pulmonary**	purson with AIDS	
Pullmotor	**pulmotor**		**person with AIDS**
pullpa	**pulpa****	purtussis	**pertussis**
pullp chamber	**pulp chamber**	purveous	**pervious****
pullpel	**pulpal****	puss	**pus**
pullse rate	**pulse rate**	pussbasin	**pus basin**
pullses	**pulses**	pusse	**pus**
pulmanary embolism		pusstuler	**pustular**
	pulmonary embolism	pustyool	**pustule**
pulmenery artery		pustyulant	**pustulant**
	pulmonary artery	pwasson	**Poisson****
pulminnary function test		pyacyanase	**pyocyanase**
	pulmonary function test	pyageens	**pyogenes****
pulmonnic valve disease		pyal	**pial****
	pulmonic valve disease	pyejens	**pyogens****
pulmunary vane	**pulmonary vein**	pyell- (pre)	**pyel-**
pulp cannal	**pulp canal**	pyello- (pre)	**pyelo-**
pulpil	**pulpal****	pyelorus	**pylorus**
pulpp	**pulp****	pyeramidon	**pyramidon**
pulsashun	**pulsation**	pyeyouria	**pyuria**
puls pressure	**pulse pressure**	pyles	**piles**
pulssis	**pulsus**	pylography	**pyelography**
puncktim	**punctum**	pyoobis	**pubis****
punktate	**punctate**	pyoobs	**pubes****
punkture	**puncture**	pyoor- (pre)	**puer-**
punsh	**punch****	pyosallpinks	**pyosalpinx**
pupall	**pupal**	pyotee	**peyote**
pupilae	**pupillae**	pyre- (pre)	**pyr-**
pupul	**pupil****	pyrectick	**pyrectic****
pur	**purr****	pyreo- (pre)	**pyro-**
purerpurer	**purupura****	pyrexxiel	**pyrexial****
purgonal	**Pergonal**	pyroertotherapy	**pyroretotherapy**
puripheral	**peripheral**	pyroll	**pyrrole**
puritic rash	**pruritic rash**	pytocin	**Pitocin**
purje	**purge**	pyuberty	**puberty**
purmeible	**permeable**	pyure	**pure****
purperal fever	**puerperal fever**	pyure- (pre)	**puer-**
purperium	**puerperium**	pyurine	**purine**
purple infection		pyurulent	**purulent**
	puerperal infection	pyutressence	**putrescence**

Q

Incorrect	Correct	Incorrect	Correct
qrs complex	**QRS complex**	quadrait lobe	**quadrate lobe**
qt tinterval	**Q-T interval**	quadralaterel	**quadrilateral**

Incorrect	Correct	Incorrect	Correct
quadraseps	**quadriceps**	Quewave	**Q wave**
quadrent	**quadrant**	quickning	**quickening**
Qualude	**Quaalude**	quiesent	**quiescent**
quantatative	**quantitative**	quincy	**quinsy**
quardri- (pre)	**quadri-**	quinicrine	**quinacrine**
quarenteen	**quarantine**	quoshant	**quotient**
quasia	**quassia**	QV	**qv**
quatenary ammonia compounds		qwackery	**quackery**
	quarternary ammonia compounds	qwantety	**quantity**
		qwinidine	**quinidine**
Que fever	**Q fever**	qwink	**Quincke****
querelent	**querulent**	qwintuplet	**quintuplet**

R

Incorrect	Correct	Incorrect	Correct
rabbet	**rabbit****	radyoisotope	**radioisotope**
rabbid	**rabid****	raediation sickness	
rabd/o- (pre)	**rhabd/o-**		**radiation sickness**
rabees	**rabies**	raediotherepy	**radiotherapy**
rabit test	**rabbit test**	rafanose	**raffinose****
rach	**rash**	rafinace	**raffinase****
radacal	**radical****	-rafy (suff)	**-rhaphy**
raddeography	**radiography**	-rage (suff)	**-rrhage**
raddical mastectomy		-ragia (suff)	**-rrhagia**
	radical mastectomy	raile	**rale**
raddikle	**radicle****	Rainaud's disease	
raddiotherapist	**radiotherapist**		**Raynaud's disease**
rade/o- (pre)	**radi/o-**	raiz	**raze****
radeal nerve	**radial nerve**	raize	**raise****
radeation	**radiation**	raki/o- (pre)	**rachi/o-**
radeo knife	**radio knife**	rammi	**rami**
radeum therapy	**radium therapy**	rammnose	**rhamnose****
radiactive	**radioactive**	rammose	**ramose****
radialogy	**radiologist**	*Ramnuss*	***Rhamnus*****
radicks	**radix**	rappid eye movement sleep	
radidontist	**radiodontist**		**rapid eye movement sleep**
radikal treatment	**radical treatment**	rashionalization	**rationalization**
radiofarmaceuticals		rashon	**ration****
	radiopharmaceuticals	rasse	**race**
radioggrapher	**radiographer**	*Rawolfia* derivative	
radiolajist	**radiologist**		***Rauwolfia* derivative**
radioopak substance	**radiopaque**	raydiation keratotomy	
radiuss	**radius**		**radiation keratotomy**
radyation therapy		rayes	**rays****
	radiation therapy	raymus	**ramus****

Incorrect	Correct
raysheo	ratio
rayson	rasion**
Ray's syndrome	Reye's syndrome
-rea (suff)	-rrhea
reachional bloc	regional block
reacktivity	reactivity
reactiv hiporemia	reactive hyperemia
read blood count	red blood count
readundent	redundant
reaktion formation	reaction formation
re-atachment	reattachment
reccomended dietary allowance	recommended dietary allowance
recepter potential	receptor potential
reckerd	record**
recktum	rectum
recommbination	recombination
re-construcktion	reconstruction
recooperasion	recuperation
recrutement	recruitment
rectel thermometer	rectal thermometer
rectes femoris	rectus femoris
rectis abdominus	rectus abdominus
rectoseal	rectocele
re-cumbant	recumbent
recurence	recurrence
red current jelly sputum	red currant jelly sputum
redd blood cell	red blood cell
red mussel fibers	red muscle fibers
reduktion	reduction
redused hemoglobin	reduced hemoglobin
ree- (pre)	re- **
reeactive disorder	reactive disorder
reeagent	reagent**
reecess	recess**
reecessive trait	recessive trait
reeconstructive surgery	reconstructive surgery
reecurent	recurrent
Reed method	Read method
reeferred pain	referred pain
reeffer	reefer**

Incorrect	Correct
reeflekts	reflects**
reeflex ark	reflex arc
reegression	regression
reejiones	regiones
reel anxiety	real anxiety
reelapsing fever	relapsing fever
reelaxed pelvic flore	relaxed pelvic floor
reembursement	reimbursement
reemission	remission
reenal	renal
reenforsement	reinforcement
reepression	repression
reesection	resection
reesipricle	reciprocal
reesponse	response
Reesus factor	rhesus factor
reet	rete
reetardation	retardation
reeticulosis	reticulosis
reetinopathy	retinopathy
reetraction sign	retraction sign
reet testis	rete testis
reeverse tolerance	reverse tolerance
referr	refer**
refferance	reference
refferral	referral
refleks	reflex**
refracksion	refraction
refraktery period	refractory period
re-fraktured	refractured
refuzal	refusal
regection	rejection
regeeme	regime
regerjitant essophagitis	regurgitant esophagitis
regerjtation	regurgitation
regestered nurse	registered nurse
reggio	regio**
reguler rithim	regular rhythm
rehabbilitation	rehabilitation
rehabillitation medicine	rehabilitation medicine
rejimen	regimen
rejun	region**
rekombinant DNA	recombinant DNA

Incorrect	Correct
rekovry room	recovery room
rekroodescence	recrudescence
rekt/o- (pre)	rect/o-
rektovaginal examination	
	rectovaginal examination
relacksent	relaxant
relaksation releef	relaxation relief
relaps	relapse
relavant	relevant**
releef	relief**
releese	release
releive	relieve**
reletive	relative
relitive refractory period	
	relative refractory period
remidy	remedy
remitent fever	remittant fever
remm sleep	REM sleep
remoovel	removal
renall colicretinitis pigmentosa	
	renal colicretinitis pigmentosa
rene- (pre)	reni-
renel pellvis	renal pelvis
renen	renin**
reneo- (pre)	renio-
renil calculus	renal calculus
reninn	rennin**
rentgeno- (pre)	roentgeno-
rentgenscope	roentgenoscope
rentjenography	roentgenography
reo- (pre)	rheo-
reparetive	reparative
repawtible disease	
	reportable disease
repettitive	repetitive
replasement therapy	
	replacement therapy
repraduktive system	
	reproductive system
rescent	recent
resektascope	resectoscope
reseption	reception
reseptive	receptive
reseptor	receptor
resession	recession
resessis	recessus**
residyal volume	residual volume
resipiant	recipient

Incorrect	Correct
resisstanse	resistance
resourcinol	resorcinol
resparatory quotient	
	respiratory quotient
resparometer	respirometer
resperation	respiration
resperratory distress syndrome	
	respiratory distress syndrome
respiritory arest	respiratory arrest
respirratory alkalosis	
	respiratory alkalosis
respitory	respiratory**
respratorry acidosis	
	respiratory acidosis
resserpine	reserpine
ressesive	recessive
resspirator	respirator
resspratory	respiratory
resst home	rest home
ressting memmbrane potential	
	resting membrane potential
ressussitator	resuscitator
restraynt	restraint
restriksion	restriction
resurch	research
resussitasion	resuscitation
retale customer	retail customer
retayned	retained
retayner	retainer
retension	retention
retergrade	retrograde
reteroflexed	retroflexed
reterovirus	retrovirus
reterspective	retrospective
reterspective billing	
	retrospective billing
retickulem	reticulum
retikuler	reticular
retna	retina**
retrackter	retractor
retraviral	retroviral
retreperitoneal	retroperitoneal
retrevirus inhibitor	
	retrovirus inhibitor
retrevurted uterus	
	retroverted uterus
retroeverted	retroverted
retrowsternel	retrosternal

Incorrect	Correct
rettarded	**retarded**
rettin/o- (pre)	**retin/o-**
rettin-A	**Retin-A****
rettinitis	**retinitis**
rettravirus	**retrovirus**
rettro- (pre)	**retro-**
rettrovirous	**retrovirus**
reu	**rue****
reumatic heart disease	
	rheumatic heart disease
revaskelerization	**revascularization**
reverced	**reversed**
revursion	**reversion**
revvalant	**revellent****
revvalution	**revolution**
Reyy's	**Reye's****
rezadent	**resident**
rezentment	**resentment**
reziduel	**residual****
rezins	**resins**
rezistent	**resistant**
rezonnense	**resonance**
rezult	**result**
rezzado	**residue****
rezzevwar	**reservoir**
RH	**Rh****
rhee	**rhe****
Rh faktor	**Rh factor**
rhonncheal	
	rhonchal or **rhonchial****
rhoom	**rheum****
rhumatology	**rheumatology**
rhyetidectomy	**rhytidectomy**
rhyn/o- (pre)	**rhin/o-**
ribanucleic acid	**ribonucleic acid**
ribb	**rib**
rib beeding	**rib beading**
ribboflavin	**riboflavin**
ribbose	**ribose**
ribnuclease	**ribonuclease**
ribone mussles	**ribbon muscles**
ribossome	**ribosome**
Riccord	**Ricord****
ricetsia	**rickettsiae**
Richardson Vicks	
	Richardson Vicks
ricketshial diseases	
	rickettsial diseases

Incorrect	Correct
ridjed	**ridged****
rigger mortus	**rigor mortis**
righter's cramp	**writer's cramp**
rij	**ridge**
rijid	**rigid****
rijidity of muscles	
	rigidity of muscles
rijjid	**rigid****
rikets	**rickets****
riktus	**rictus**
rinelith	**rhinolith**
ring finnger	**ring finger**
ring kromosome	**ring chromosome**
ringwurm	**ringworm**
rinitis	**rhinitis**
rinkling	**wrinkling**
rino- (pre)	**rhino-**
rinoplasty	**rhinoplasty**
risq	**risk**
rist	**wrist**
rist bone	**wrist bone**
rite ventricle	**right ventricle**
rithing	**writhing**
rithmical tremmer	
	rhythmical tremor
rithmic korea	**rhythmic chorea**
rithm method	**rhythm method**
ritten orders	**written orders**
rizotomy	**rhizotomy**
Robinns	**Robins**
Rochel powders	**Rochelle powders**
Rockey Mountin spotted fever	
	Rocky Mountain spotted fever
rod- (pre)	**rhod-**
rodd	**rod**
rodo- (pre)	**rhodo-**
Rolet	**Rollet****
Rolett	**Rollett****
Rollaids	**Rolaids**
Rollfing	**rolfing**
romboid	**rhomboid**
roncal	**rhonchal**
ronchus	**rhonchus**
roncus	**rhoncus**
ronger	**rongeur**
rongful death	**wrongful death**
roo	**Roux****
roomatism	**rheumatism**

Incorrect	Correct
roote	**root****
Rorshak	**Rorschach**
Roshe	**Roche**
rotater cuf	**rotator cuff**
rotovirus	**rotavirus**
roufage	**roughage**
rouff endoplasmic reticulum .... **rough endoplasmic reticulum**	
rouns	**rounds**
rouwolfia	**rauwolfia**
rowtation	**rotation**
rowtery	**rotary**
rowtetory	**rotatory**
rozacea	**rosacea**
rozeola	**roseola****
rubbor	**rubber****
rubela	**rubella****
ruber gloves	**rubber gloves**
rubifacient	**rubefacient**
rubine	**rubin**
Rubinn	**Rubin**
rubiola	**rubeola****
rubor	**ruber****

Incorrect	Correct
rubore	**rubor****
RUE-486	**RU-486**
ruegal	**rugal**
ruematoid arthritis .... **rheumatoid arthritis**	
rueteen	**routine**
ruffage	**roughage**
ruff endoplasmic reticulum .... **rough endoplasmic reticulum**	
rugay	**rugae**
ruggal	**rugal**
rumatic fever	**rheumatic fever**
runing	**running**
runy nose	**runny nose**
rupcher	**rupture**
rupchured disk	**ruptured disc**
Russ	**Ross**
russty sputum	**rusty sputum**
rute canal	**root canal**
rute sheeth	**root sheath**
ryneck	**wryneck**
rynolight	**rhinolith**
rynorea	**rhinorrhea**

S

Incorrect	Correct
sabbaceous sist	**sebaceous cyst**
Sabbin vaccine	**Sabin vaccine**
saccs	**sacs****
sacherated fat	**saturated fat**
sachrifying enzyme .... **saccharifying enzyme**	
sachs	**Sachs****
sachuration	**saturation**
sackarase	**saccharase**
sackaride group	**saccharide group**
sackrum	**sacrum**
sackulated aneurism .... **sacculated aneurysm**	
sacrecoccygeal	**sacrococcygeal**
sacregenital fold	**sacrogenital fold**
sacrel vertebrae	**sacral vertebrae**
sacril nerve	**sacral nerve**
sacrin	**saccharin****
sacule	**saccule****

Incorrect	Correct
sacyule	**sacculi****
sadamasokism	**sadomasochism**
saddel block	**saddle block**
sadeism	**sadism**
saif	**safe**
saint vitustance	**Saint Vitus' Dance**
saiv	**save****
sajital sinus	**sagittal sinus**
sakerine	**saccharine****
sakr/o- (pre)	**sacr/o-**
sakroiliac	**sacroiliac**
sakrose	**saccharose**
sakule	**saccule****
salavery amilase	**salivary amylase**
salean	**saline**
saliclic asid	**salicylic acid**
sall amoniac	**sal ammoniac**
sallisylic acid	**salicylic acid**
sallivary glands	**salivary glands**

Incorrect	Correct	Incorrect	Correct
sallmine	**salmine**	scafoid	**scaphoid**
Sallmonela	*Salmonella*	scail	**scale**
Sallol	**salol**	scalled	**scald**
sallping- (pre)	**salping-**	scallpel	**scalpel**
sallpingectomy	**salpingectomy**	scann	**scan**
sallpingo- (pre)	**salpingo-**	scappala	**scapula****
sallpingo-ophorectomy		scappul/o- (pre)	**scapul/o-**
	salpingo-oophorectomy	scarlitina	**scarlatina**
salmenella	**salmonella**	scarr	**scar****
salpinggotomy	**salapingotomy**	scarrlet fever	**scarlet fever**
salpinjitis	**salpingitis**	scaybees	**scabies**
saltz	**salts**	scaylene	**scalene**
samonella poisoning		scayler	**scaler**
	salmonella poisoning	sceletal	**skeletal**
sampel	**sample**	sceleton	**skeleton**
sanatery napkin	**sanitary napkin**	Scenters for Disease Control	
sanatorium	**sanitorium**		**Centers for Disease Control**
sanattory	**sanatory****	scervy	**scurvy**
sanfly fever	**sandfly fever**	schadow cell	**shadow cell**
sangin/o- (pre)	**sanguin/o-**	schank	**shank**
sangwineous		scharp pane	**sharp pain**
	sanguineous or **sanguinous**	schigella	**shigella**
sanitive	**sanative**	schisokenesis	**schizokinesis**
Sanndoz	**Sandoz**	schitsoid personality	
sannetary	**sanitary****		**schizoid personality**
sannitory	**sanatory****	schizofrenic patient	
Sannofi Winthrop	**Sanofi Winthrop**		**schizophrenic patient**
saper/o- (pre)	**sapr/o-**	schort pulss	**short pulse**
saporphyte	**saprophyte**	schoulder blade	**shoulder blade**
sarcamer	**sarcomere**	schunt	**shunt**
sarck- (pre)	**sarc-**	scipped beet	**skipped beat**
sarko- (pre)	**sarco-**	scizofrenia	**schizophrenia**
sarkoma	**sarcoma**	sckerge	**scourge**
sarkosin	**sarcosine**	sclarosed	**sclerosed**
sarrcoid	**sarcoid**	sclerr/o- (pre)	**scler/o-**
sarrtorius	**sartorius**	sclerroderma	**scleroderma**
sarsina	**sarcina**	-sclerrosis (suff)	**-sclerosis**
sasafras	**sassafras**	sclerrus	**sclerous****
satessfactorly	**satisfactorily**	sclerus tishues	**sclerous tissues**
satiryasis	**satyriasis**	sclirectomy	**sclerectomy**
sattelite	**satellite**	scoar	**score**
sattisfactery	**satisfactory**	scoleosis	**scoliosis**
Sauk vaccine	**Salk vaccine**	scoppolamine	**scopolamine**
sav	**salve****	-scoppy (suff)	**-scopy**
Saybin vaccine	**Sabin vaccine**	scrach	**scratch**
sayline solution	**saline solution**	scrayping	**scraping**
scabasides	**scabicides**	screan	**screen**
scabb	**scab**	screning	**screening**

Incorrect	Correct	Incorrect	Correct
scroetim	**scrotum**	seel	**seal*** *
scrofelous	**scrofulous**	seemen	**semen*** *
scroffula	**scrofula**	seemless	**seamless**
scrowtle	**scrotal**	seemon	**Semon*** *
scrubb suit	**scrub suit**	seenile	**senile**
scrue	**screw**	seequence pyelogram	
scull	**skull**		**sequence pyelogram**
scurge	**scourge**	seerim	**serum*** *
seal- (pre)	**sial-**	seeropositivity	**seropositivity**
sealo- (pre)	**sialo-**	seerum	**serum*** *
seamen	**semen*** *	seesickness	**seasickness**
seasarean section	**Cesarean section**	seezonal affective disorder	
seasure	**seizure**		**seasonal affective disorder**
sebareic dermatitis		seezure	**seizure**
	seborrheic dermatitis	seggmentation	**segmentation**
sebashous gland	**sebaceous gland**	seggmented	**segmented**
sebberea	**seborrhea**	seggmentim	**segmentum**
seberhea	**seborrhea**	segmentle	**segmental**
secand-degree burn		segragation	**segregation**
	second-degree burn	Seidenham's chorea	
Secconal	**Seconal**		**Sydenham's chorea**
secction	**section**	seight	**sight*** *
secks-limited	**sex-limited**	sekondary care	**secondary care**
seckter irridectomy		sekreta	**secreta*** *
	sector iridectomy	sekshally transmitted disease	
secreetion	**secretion*** *		**sexually transmitted disease**
secritory vessicles	**secretory vesicles**	seksual dimorphism	
secs change operation			**sexual dimorphism**
	sex change operation	sektion	**section**
secum	**cecum**	sekwential oral contraceptives	
seddetive	**sedative**		**sequential oral contraceptives**
sedd rate	**SED rate**	sela	**sella*** *
sedementation rate		-selaphasia (suff)	**-pselaphesia**
	sedimentation rate	seler	**sellar*** *
seditive	**sedative**	self infection	**self-infection**
Seeba	**Ciba**	self-viktimization	**self-victimization**
seebum	**sebum**	seliac disease	**celiac disease**
seecobarbital sodium		sell	**cell*** *
	secobarbital sodium	sell division	**cell division**
seecreet	**secrete*** *	sellective arteriography	
seecretin	**secretin*** *		**selective arteriography**
SEECUS	**SIECUS**	sellf-treatment	**self-treatment**
seedation	**sedation**	sellpingopalatine fold	
see gull mermer	**seagull murmur**		**salpingopalatine fold**
seeing ey dog	**seeing eye dog**	sells	**cells**
seek- (pre)	**cec-**	sellulite reduction	**cellulite reduction**
seeko- (pre)	**ceco-**	sellulitis	**cellulitis**
seekretion	**secretion*** *	sellulose	**cellulose**

Incorrect	Correct
seltser	**seltzer**
seme- (pre)	**semi-**
semecircular canal	
	semicircular canal
seme-lunar	**semilunar**
semenal vesicle	**seminal vesicle**
semenifferous tubules	
	seminiferous tubules
sementum	**cementum**
semeology ...	**semeiology** or **semiology**
semmin/o- (pre)	**semin/o-**
semminal vesicle	**seminal vesicle**
semmi-permeable membrane	
	semipermeable membrane
semyotics	**semeiotics** or **semiotics**
sena	**senna**
sence organs	**sense organs**
sencer	**censor****
sencibility	**sensibility**
sencitivity	**sensitivity**
sencitization	**sensitization**
senessence	**senescence**
senillity	**senility**
sennile sychosis	**senile psychosis**
sennilis	**senilis**
sennsetive	**sensitive**
senser	**sensor****
sensetive	**sensitive**
sensry receptors	**sensory receptors**
sensus	**census****
Senters for Disease Control	
	Centers for Disease Control
-sentesis (suff)	**-centesis**
sentinnel polip	**sentinel polyp**
sentral nervous system	
	central nervous system
sentral thurmoreceptors	
	central thermoreceptors
sentrioles	**centrioles**
sentromere	**centromere**
sentrum	**centrum**
seperate pockets of pus	
	separate pockets of pus
seperating sore	**separating saw**
seperation	**separation**
sephalo- (pre)	**cephalo-**
sepparation	**separation**
seppsis	**sepsis**

Incorrect	Correct
sepptic	**septic**
sepsus	**sepsis**
septesemia	**septicemia**
septik abortion	**septic abortion**
septim	**septum**
septisemic meningitis	
	septicemic meningitis
septle deviation	**septal deviation**
serated	**serrated****
seratherapy	**serotherapy**
sereaction	**seroreaction**
serebral	**cerebral**
serebrum	**cerebrum****
serface	**surface**
serfers not	**surfer's knot**
Sergeon General	**Surgeon General**
serim transfusion	
	serum transfusion
Serle	**Searle**
seroe- (pre)	**sero-**
seroenegativity	**seronegativity**
serollgy	**serology**
serrebelum	**cerebellum****
serrebrospinal fever	
	cerebrospinal fever
serrine	**serine**
serrious	**serious****
serrology	**serology**
serrotonin	**serotonin**
serroundings	**surroundings**
serrum albumin	**serum albumin**
serrum globulin	**serum globulin**
serumen	**cerumen****
servalance	**surveillance**
servay	**survey**
servic- (pre)	**cervic-**
servical cap	**cervical cap**
servici- (pre)	**cervici-**
servival	**survival**
servucal vertebray	
	cervical vertebrae
sesion	**session**
sessation	**cessation**
seudopregnancy	**pseudopregnancy**
seveer	**severe**
severrity	**severity**
sex-kromatin	**sex chromatin**
sex kromosome	**sex chromosome**

Incorrect	Correct	Incorrect	Correct

sex-linkege .... **sex-linkage**
sexx reassignment surgery ....
.... **sex reassignment surgery**
sfear .... **sphere**
sfenoid .... **sphenoid**
sfenoidal .... **sphenoidal**
sferical abberation ....
.... **spherical aberration**
sferoid joynt .... **spheroid joint**
sfigmograph .... **sphygmograph**
sfygmommeter .... **sphygmometer****
shafft .... **shaft**
shaiking palcy .... **shaking palsy**
shalow breething .... **shallow breathing**
shancre .... **chancre****
shawt wave diathermy machine ......
.... **shortwave diathermy machine**
sheatsu .... **Shiatsu**
sheef .... **sheaf****
sheeld .... **shield**
sheeth .... **sheath****
Shering .... **Schering**
shethe .... **sheathe****
shifshin splint .... **shift-shin splint**
Shiggela .... *Shigella*
shiggelosis .... **shigellosis**
shingels .... **shingles**
shinn bone .... **shinbone**
shist/o- (pre) .... **schist/o-**
shivvers .... **shivers**
shmutz piorea ...... **Schmutz pyorrhea**
shoc .... **shock**
shody .... **shoddy****
shok reaction .... **shock reaction**
sholder .... **shoulder**
shook therapy .... **shock therapy**
shortning reaction ....
.... **shortening reaction**
shott .... **shot**
shottee .... **shotty****
shuger .... **sugar**
shulltz .... **Schultz**
shullze .... **Schultze**
Shwann cells .... **Schwann's cells**
siano- (pre) .... **cyano-**
sibb .... **sib**
sibbling .... **sibling**
sic bay .... **sick bay**

sichiatric .... **psychiatric**
sichogenic .... **psychogenic**
sichology .... **psychology**
sichophisiological ....
.... **psychophysiological**
sichophysiology ..... **psychophysiology**
sichosexual disorder ....
.... **psychosexual disorder**
sichosomatic illness ....
.... **psychosomatic illness**
sichotherapeutic drugs ....
.... **psychotherapeutic drugs**
sichotherapist .... **psychotherapist**
sickbed .... **sick bed**
sickelcell .... **sickle-cell**
sickel skaler .... **sickle scaler**
sickiatry .... **psychiatry**
siclecell anemia .... **sickle-cell anemia**
sicness .... **sickness**
sicosis .... **sycosis****
-sidal (suff) .... **-cidal**
sidder/o- (pre) .... **sider/o-**
sidds .... **SIDS**
sideffect .... **side effect**
sidovudine .... **zidovudine**
Siedlitz powders ..... **Seidlitz powders**
sientific .... **scientific**
siffilis .... **syphilis**
siggmoid colon .... **sigmoid colon**
sightoplasm .... **cytoplasm**
signe .... **sign****
signitis .... **sinusitis**
sign wave .... **sine wave**
sikatrix .... **cicatrix**
sikelothymic personality ....
.... **cyclothymic personality**
sikosensory disturbance ....
.... **psychosensory disturbance**
sikotic .... **psychotic**
sik room .... **sick room**
silacone .... **silicone****
silacosis .... **silicosis**
silc suchure .... **silk suture**
silhewette .... **silhouette**
silikone-jel implant ....
.... **silicone-gel implant**
sillia .... **cilia**
sillicon .... **silicon****

84

sillicone implant ...... **silicone implant**
sillik/o- (pre)........................ **silic/o-**
sillium .... **cilium****
sillium seed .... **psyllium seed**
sillver protein .... **silver protein**
silocin .... **psilocin**
silosis .... **psilosis**
silvian .... **sylvian**
sim- (pre) ....**sym-**
simbiosus .... **symbiosis**
Simese twins .... **Siamese twins**
simetry .... **symmetry**
simfisis .... **symphysis**
simielogy ... **semeiology or semiology**
simmetrical .... **symmetrical**
simmetry .... **symmetry**
simmple fracture....... **simple fracture**
simmulate .... **simulate****
simpatholytic .... **sympatholytic**
simpethetic .... **sympathetic**
simphysis .... **symphysis**
simplecks .... **simplex**
simptomatic .... **symptomatic**
simptomatology ...... **symptomatology**
simtom .... **symptom**
simyalate .... **simulate****
sin- (pre) .... **cin-**
sinapse .... **synapse****
sinchronous .... **synchronous**
sincope .... **syncope**
sindezm/o- (pre) .... **syndesm/o-**
sindrome .... **syndrome**
sinergism .... **synergism**
sinesents .... **senescence**
singel foton emission computed
tomography ....
.... **single photon emission
computed tomography**
singel hairlip .... **single harelip**
singulitus .... **singultus**
sinicitis .... **sinusitis**
sinis .... **sinus****
sinn- (pre) ....**syn-**
sinnerjy .... **synergy**
sinnthetic .... **synthetic**
sino- (pre) .... **cino-**
sinotosis .... **synotosis**
sinotrial node .... **sinoatrial node**

sinovial .... **synovial**
sinovial capsule .... **synovial capsule**
Sintex .... **Syntex**
sinthesis .... **synthesis**
sintone ....**syntone**
sinuss rhythm .... **sinus rhythm**
sinyuous .... **sinuous****
siphilis .... **syphilis**
siphilitic .... **syphilitic**
sirebral hemorrhage ....
.... **cerebral hemorrhage**
sirfactant .... **surfactant**
sirkumcision .... **circumcision**
sirogate mother ...... **surrogate mother**
sirosa .... **serosa**
sirosis .... **cirrhosis**
sirous .... **scirrhous****
sirrebrovascular accident ....
.... **cerebrovascular accident**
sirrup of ipecac .... **syrup of ipecac**
Sirtoli cell .... **Sertoli's cell**
sirus .... **scirrhus****
sirynge .... **syringe**
sischosiss .... **sycosis****
sisst .... **cyst**
sisstemic circulation ....
.... **systemic circulation**
sisstitis .... **cystitis**
sisstoscopy .... **cystoscopy**
sist- (pre) .... **cyst-**
sistectomy .... **cystectomy**
sistem .... **system**
sistemic .... **systemic**
sisti- (pre) .... **cysti-**
sistic duck .... **cystic duct**
sistic fibrosis .... **cystic fibrosis**
sistine .... **cystine**
sisto- (pre) .... **cysto-**
sistography .... **cystography**
sistole .... **systole**
sistoma .... **cystoma**
sistomatic .... **systematic**
sistomiasis .... **schistosomiasis**
sistoscopy ....**cystoscopy**
sitakrome .... **cytochrome**
sitameggalovirus ...... **cytomegalovirus**
sitchuation .... **situation**
-site (suff) ....**-cyte****

Incorrect	Correct
siteology	sitology**
siteprotective	cytoprotective
sitescope	cytoscope
sito- (pre)	cyto-
sitogenetics	cytogenetics
sitokinesis	cytokinesis
sitomegalovirus	cytomegalovirus
sitoplasm	cytoplasm
sitosine	cytosine
sitoxin	cytotoxin
sitric acid cycle	citric acid cycle
sits bath	sitz bath
sitte- (pre)	cyt-
sittoglobulin	cytoglobulin
situashonal psichosis	situational psychosis
sizzers	scissors
skabbing	scabbing
skabetic infection	scabetic infection
Skains ducts	Skene's ducts
skale	scale
skalene	scalene
skalp	scalp
skapuler	scapular**
skatoma	scatoma**
skelletal	skeletal
skelleton	skeleton
skineitis	skenitis
Skiner	Skinner
skin iruption	skin eruption
skinn	skin
skinngraft	skin graft
skirus	scirrhus**
-skisis (suff)	-schisis
skoliosis	scoliosis
skiso- (pre)	schizo-
skitso- (pre)	schizo-
skizatypal personality	schizotypal personality
skizoid	schizoid
skizophrenic payshent	schizophrenic patient
skizothymia	schizothymia
sklera	sclera
sklerae	sclerae
skleral	scleral

Incorrect	Correct
skleral cressent	scleral crescent
sklerictoridectomy	sclerectoiridectomy
sklerosis	sclerosis
sklerro- (pre)	sclero-
sklerrose	sclerose**
skoetoma	scotoma**
skoop	scoop
-skop (suff)	-scope
-skopic (suff)	-scopic
skopolamine	scopolamine
skopp/o- (pre)	scop/o-
skore	score
skottoma	scotoma**
skrape	scrape
skraping	scraping
skratch	scratch
skratch test	scratch test
skreen	screen
skrot/o- (pre)	scrot/o-
skrotal	scrotal
skrotim	scrotum
skrub nurse	scrub nurse
skrub-suit	scrub suit
skul	skull
skurf	scurf
skurge	scourge
skwamous cell	squamous cell
skwamus cell	squamous cell
skwint	squint
slach	slash
sleap and dreams	sleep and dreams
sleapping sickness	sleeping sickness
slepe walking	sleepwalking
sleping pill	sleeping pill
slidding-filament mechanism	sliding-filament mechanism
slinng	sling
slipt disk	slipped disc
slise	slice
slitely	slightly
sliva	saliva
sloe-wave sleep	slow-wave sleep
sluf	slough
slugish reaction	sluggish reaction
slured speech	slurred speech

Incorrect	Correct
smal intestine	**small intestine**
smallpocks	**smallpox**
smalpox	**smallpox**
smegna	**smegma**
smeling salts	**smelling salts**
smere	**smear**
Smith Klein Beecham ...	**SmithKline Beecham**
smoothe endoplasmic reticulum ...	**smooth endoplasmic reticulum**
smuve mussles	**smooth muscles**
snair	**snare**
snale fever	**snail fever**
sneaze	**sneeze**
sneese	**sneeze**
sniffel	**sniffle**
snifle	**sniffle**
snorr	**snore**
soas	**psoas**
sockette	**socket**
soddium amabarbital ...	**sodium amobarbital**
soddium salycylate	**sodium salicylate**
sodeum	**sodium**
sodium fosphate ..	**sodium phosphate**
sodium hidroxide ...	**sodium hydroxide**
sodiumm hipochlorite ...	**sodium hypochlorite**
sodyim bromide	**sodium bromide**
soedium bicarbonate ...	**sodium bicarbonate**
soel	**sole****
soematic receptor	**somatic receptor**
sof tissue damage ...	**soft tissue damage**
soft pallate	**soft palate**
soft tishue	**soft tissue**
soler plexus	**solar plexus**
soll	**sol****
sollar plexus	**solar plexus**
sollu	**soul****
solleus	**soleus**
sollitery nodule	**solitary nodule**
solluable insulen	**soluble insulin**
sollution	**solution**
somambulism	**somnambulism**

Incorrect	Correct
somataform disorder ...	**somatoform disorder**
somatatropinn	**somatotropin**
somatejenic sychosomatic disorder ...	**somatogenic psychosomatic disorder**
somattoplazm	**somatoplasm**
-somia (suff)	**-somia**
somitization reaction ...	**somatization disorder**
somma	**soma****
sommat/o- (pre)	**somat/o-**
sommatic delusion ...	**somatic delusion**
sommatropic hormoan ...	**somatotropic hormone**
sommi- (pre)	**somni-**
sonagram	**sonogram**
sonn/o- (pre)	**son/o-**
soofle	**souffle**
soopine	**supine**
soore	**soor****
soparific	**soporific**
sopporific	**soporific**
sora	**psora**
sorasis	**psoriasis**
sorr	**sore****
sorrbose	**sorbose**
soshalized medicine ...	**socialized medicine**
sosheopath	**sociopath**
soshil sychology	**social psychology**
sosiopath	**sociopath**
-sowmia (suff)	**-somia**
sownd	**sound**
Spannish fly	**Spanish fly**
spase	**space**
spase meddicine	**space medicine**
spashial	**spatial****
spasial summation ...	**spatial summation**
spasim	**spasm**
spassia	**spatia****
spasstic colon	**spastic colon**
spastick contracters ...	**spastic contractures**

spastissity .... **spasticity**
spattula .... **spatula**
-spazim (suff) .... **-spasm**
spazm .... **spasm**
spazmodic .... **spasmodic**
speach disorders ..... **speech disorders**
specculum ....**speculum**
specemin bottle .... **specimen bottle**
speciallist .... **specialist**
speciffic dinamic action ....
.... **specific dynamic action**
speeshez .... **species**
speetch disfunction ....
.... **speech dysfunction**
spektinomisin .... **spectinomycin**
spel .... **spell**
spermasidal jelly ..... **spermicidal jelly**
spermisside .... **spermicide**
spermitajenesis .... **spermatogenesis**
spermmatozone .... **spermatozoon**
sperrmatic cord .... **spermatic cord**
sperrmatt/o- (pre) .... **spermat/o-**
speshalist .... **specialist**
spessificity .... **specificity**
spessimin .... **specimen**
sphigmanometer ....
.... **sphygmomanometer****
sphinkter .... **sphincter**
spiccule .... **spicule****
spicke pattern .... **spike pattern**
spickuler .... **spicula****
spike of the shoulder ....
.... **spica of the shoulder**
spikking disrithmia ....
.... **spiking dysrhythmia**
spilt protein .... **spilled protein**
spinall cored .... **spinal cord**
Spinbarkite .... **spinnbarkeit**
spindel fibers .... **spindle fibers**
spinil column .... **spinal column**
spinill menengitis ....
.... **spinal meningitis**
spinna bifida .... **spina bifida**
spinndle .... **spindle**
spiragraff .... **spirograph**
spirall .... **spiral**
spirm .... **sperm**
spirokete .... **spirochete**

spirrillim .... **spirillum**
spirrits of camfer ....
.... **spirits of camphor**
splanshnic .... **splanchnic**
splean .... **spleen**
splen/o- (pre) .... **splen/o-**
splennic .... **splenic**
splintt .... **splint**
splising .... **splicing**
spliting .... **splitting**
split pursonality .... **split personality**
splitt brane .... **split brain**
spondilitis .... **spondylitis**
spondilossis .... **spondylosis**
sponjy bone .... **spongy bone**
sponndil/o- (pre) .... **spondyl/o-**
sponntaneous abortion ....
.... **spontaneous abortion**
spore/i/o- (pre) .... **spor/i/o-**
sporr .... **spore**
sporradic .... **sporadic**
sporrts medisine .... **sports medicine**
spoted fever .... **spotted fever**
spoting .... **spotting**
sprane .... **sprain**
sprilla .... **spirilla**
sproo .... **sprue**
spucific therapy .... **specific therapy**
spunje .... **sponge**
spurm- (pre) .... **sperm-**
spurma- (pre) .... **sperma-**
spurm count .... **sperm count**
spurmi- (pre) .... **spermi-**
spurmo- (pre) .... **spermo-**
spurr .... **spur**
sputim .... **sputum**
spynal accessory nerve ....
.... **spinal accessory nerve**
spyne .... **spine**
spyro- (pre) .... **spiro-**
spyrometer .... **spirometer**
spyutum .... **sputum**
stabeel .... **stabile****
stach .... **starch**
staf .... **staff****
Staficillin .... **Staphcillin**
stafl/o- (pre) .... **staphyl/o-**
stafylococci .... **staphylococci**

Incorrect	Correct
stait	state**
staj	stage
standerd	standard
stane	stain
staning	staining
stanstill	standstill
staphe	staph**
staphloccocus	staphylococcus
-stassis (suff)	-stasis
-state (suff)	-stat
statick	static
statt	stat**
stattus	status
stayble	stable**
staydeum	stadium
staypes	stapes
staysis	stasis
steathoskope	stethoscope
stedy state	steady state
steerile	stearoyl**
steet/o- (pre)	steat/o-
stefness	stiffness
stela	stella**
stelate	stellate
steler	stellar**
stemm	stem
stennosis	stenosis
stennt	stent
stenoclaviculer	sternoclavicular
stenotomy	sternotomy
steral saline solution	sterile saline solution
sterel	sterile**
sternel	sternal
sternim	sternum
steroyd	steroid
sterrile	sterile**
sterrility	sterility
sterrlisation	sterilization
sterroid	steroid
sterrol	sterol**
stertorous respiration	stertorous respiration
stethagraph	stethograph
stethascope	stethoscope
stethommeter	stethometer
stich	stitch
stie	sty or stye

Incorrect	Correct
stilborne	stillborn
stillbestrol	stilbestrol
stiloglossis	styloglossus
stilohyoid	stylohyoid
stimmulant	stimulant
stimmulate	stimulate**
stimmulation	stimulation
stimyalate	stimulate**
stimyalus	stimulus
stimyulent	stimulant
stirn/o- (pre)	stern/o-
stirups	stirrups
stitchs	stitches
stoan	stone
stomak pump	stomach pump
stomic	stomach
stomma	stoma**
stommat/o- (pre)	stomat/o-
stommatitis	stomatitis
stommich tube	stomach tube
-stommy or stommies (suff)	-stomy or stomies
stoole	stool
stoope	stupe**
stooper	stupor
stown	stone
strabbismus	strabismus
strabizmis	strabismus
straetum lucidum	stratum lucidum
straightjacket	straitjacket
strane	strain
stranjery	strangury
stratagy	strategy
strate	straight
stratejacket	straitjacket
stratim corneum	stratum corneum
strattegy	strategy
strattum granulosum	stratum granulosum
strauberry mark	strawberry mark
straytum germinativum	stratum germinativum
strecher	stretcher
strech marks	stretch marks
strenous exersize	strenuous exercise
strenth	strength
strepdo- (pre)	strepto-

89

Incorrect	Correct	Incorrect	Correct
strepp throat	**strep throat**	sub-aortic	**subaortic**
strepptomycin	**streptomycin**	sub-atomic	**subatomic**
streptacoccal sore throat		subb- (pre)	**sub-**
	streptococcal sore throat	subbclavian trunk	**subclavian trunk**
streptccocci	**streptococci**	subbdermel	**subdermal**
streptethrycin	**streptothricin**	subbdural	**subdural**
streptoe- (pre)	**strept/o-**	subblime	**sublime****
strepttococcis	**streptococcus**	subbmandibuler	**submandibular**
stres	**stress**	subbmucous	**submucous**
stress frakture	**stress fracture**	subbnormel	**subnormal**
stress inkontinence		subbstance abuse disorder	
	stress incontinence		**substance abuse disorder**
stress manejement		subbstanchia	**substantia****
	stress management	subbstitution therapy	
stress reakshon	**stress reaction**		**substitution therapy**
stress reeceptor	**stress receptor**	subcappusculer	**subcapsular**
stress tesst	**stress test**	subclinnical	**subclinical**
striay	**striae****	subcutticular	**subcuticular**
strichnine	**strychnine**	subcyootenous fat	**subcutaneous fat**
strickture	**stricture****	subcyutaneous	**subcutaneous**
strider	**stridor**	subdooral hematoma	
strikenyne	**strychnine**		**subdural hematoma**
stripp	**strip****	subjecktive	**subjective**
stroak	**stroke**	subklavian	**subclavian**
stroema	**stroma****	subklavicular mermer	
strok volume	**stroke volume**		**subclavicular murmur**
strommal	**stromal**	subkonshus	**subconscious**
struckture	**structure****	subkostal	**subcostal**
strukteralism	**structuralism**	sublamation	**sublimation**
strumonium	**stramonium**	sublingwil gland	**sublingual gland**
strya	**stria**	sublucksation	**subluxation**
stryated muscle	**striated muscle**	sublyne	**subline****
strype	**stripe****	submaksallary gland	
stubb	**stub**		**submaxillary gland**
stule	**stool**	submentle	**submental**
stumach ache	**stomachache**	submeted	**submitted**
stumpp	**stump**	submukosal	**submucosal**
stuntt	**stunt**	subnoremality	**subnormality**
stuper	**stupor**	substanshal	**substantial****
stureen	**sturine**	substense	**substance**
sturnokleidomastoid		substernnal	**substernal**
	sternocleidomastoid	substetution	**substitution**
sturnutation	**sternutation**	substrait	**substrate**
stuter	**stutter**	subtiln	**subtilin**
stuttring	**stuttering**	suburril heematoma	
stylett	**stylet**		**subdural hematoma**
styllomastoid	**stylomastoid**	succis	**succus****
subakute	**subacute**	suchured	**sutured**

Incorrect	Correct	Incorrect	Correct

sucidial .... **suicidal**
sucksinylsulfathiazole ....
.... **succinylsulfathiazole**
sucktion .... **suction**
Suckus Entericus ..... **succus entericus**
sucross .... **sucrose****
sud- (pre) .... **pseud-**
suddin .... **sudden**
suden infant death syndrome ....
.... **sudden infant death syndrome**
sudo- (pre) .... **pseudo-**
sudomallei .... **pseudomallei**
sudomembranous ....
.... **pseudomembranous**
sudomucineous .... **pseudomucinous**
sudoparalysis .... **pseudoparalysis**
sudotabes .... **pseudotabes**
suecrase .... **sucrase****
suema .... **summa**
sueside .... **suicide**
sufacation .... **suffocation**
suffishent .... **sufficient**
sufication .... **suffocation**
sugjestion therapy ....
.... **suggestion therapy**
sukkus .... **succuss****
sukrose .... **sucrose****
sulfammerizine .... **sulfamerazine**
sulfannethilmethane ....
.... **sulfonethylmethane**
sulfassoxazole .... **sulfisoxazole**
Sulfasuxxidine .... **Sulfasuxidine**
sulfathyizole .... **sulfathiazole**
sulfer .... **sulfur****
sulfidymethoxine ... **sulfadimethoxine**
sulfinilamide .... **sulfanilamide**
Sulfithallidine .... **Sulfathalidine**
sulfonnamide .... **sulfonamide**
sulfurpyrazine .... **sulfapyrazine**
Sulivan .... **Sullivan**
sulkus .... **sulcus**
Sullavanian theory ....
.... **Sullivanian theory**
sullfa .... **sulfa****
sullfadiazine .... **sulfadiazine**
sullfapirradine .... **sulfapyridine**
sulphaguanidine .... **sulfaguanidine**
sulpha level .... **sulfa level**

sulpho- (pre) .... **sulfo-****
suma- (pre) .... **soma-**
sumation .... **summation**
sumatosychology ....
.... **somatopsychology**
sumnolent .... **somnolent**
sunbern .... **sunburn**
sunnstroke .... **sunstroke**
supaficial infections ....
.... **superficial infections**
suparenal .... **suprarenal**
supavizer .... **supervisor**
supera- (pre) .... **supra-**
superating gastritus ....
.... **suppurating gastritis**
superation .... **suppuration**
superclaveculer .... **supraclavicular**
superenal gland ...... **suprarenal gland**
superfishal .... **superficial**
supernummery .... **supernumerary**
superorbitel .... **supraorbital**
superpateler .... **suprapatellar**
superskapuler .... **suprascapular**
supertroklear .... **supratrochlear**
superventicular .... **supraventricular**
supervition .... **supervision**
superyor .... **superior**
supireority complex ....
.... **superiority complex**
suplement .... **supplement**
suport .... **support**
suportive .... **supportive**
supository .... **suppository**
supozittory .... **suppository**
supper- (pre) .... **super-**
suppliment .... **supplement**
supprapubic .... **suprapubic**
suprafishal .... **superficial**
supresor T cell .... **suppressor T cell**
supression .... **suppression**
sur- (pre) .... **ser-**
surragncy **surrogacy**
surebral cortex .... **cerebral cortex**
surgacal dressing .... **surgical dressing**
surgecal staple .... **surgical staple**
surgicall sponge .... **surgical sponge**
surgicle mask .... **surgical mask**
surgikal gown .... **surgical gown**

Incorrect	Correct	Incorrect	Correct
surgikle needle	**surgical needle**	sychophysiological	
surgikotherapy	**surgicotherapy**		**psychophysiological**
surgisenter	**surgicenter**	sychosensary disturbence	
surgury consent form			**psychosensory disturbancc**
	surgery consent form	sychosexual disorder	
surjacal gloves	**surgical gloves**		**psychosexual disorder**
surjery	**surgery**	sychosis	**psychosis****
Surpasil	**Serpasil**	sychosomatic illness	
surragate	**surrogate**		**psychosomatic illness**
surrgical instruments		sychosomattic disorder	
	surgical instruments		**psychosomatic disorder**
surum hepetitis	**serum hepatitis**	sychotherapeutic drugs	
survical nerve	**cervical nerve**		**psychotherapeutic drugs**
suseptible	**susceptible**	sychotherapist	**psychotherapist**
suspencery	**suspensory**	sychotic	**psychotic**
suspention	**suspension**	syckobabble	**psychobabble**
suspitious	**suspicious**	syclazocine	**cyclazocine**
susseptibility	**susceptibility**	syclic AMP	**cyclic AMP**
sustaned cardiac arest		syclic GMP	**cyclic GMP**
	sustained cardiac arrest	sycloid	**cycloid**
sutcher	**suture**	syclopropane	**cyclopropane**
sutture	**suture**	sycloserine	**cycloserine**
sutyura	**sutura**	syfilis	**syphilis**
sutyure needle	**suture needle**	syfilitic	**syphilitic**
swabb	**swab**	sygmoid colon	**sigmoid colon**
swalow	**swallow**	sygmoid flexure	**sigmoid flexure**
swalowing	**swallowing**	sygmoidoscope	**sigmoidoscope**
swaybak	**swayback**	sygnificant pathology	
sweling	**swelling**		**significant pathology**
swet	**sweat**	syikotherapeutic drugs	
sweting	**sweating**		**psychotherapeutic drugs**
swett gland	**sweat gland**	syk- (pre)	**psych-**
swolen	**swollen**	syko- (pre)	**psycho-**
sy	**psi**	sykofarmacology	
syanosis	**cyanosis**		**psychopharmacology**
syatica	**sciatica**	sylent carsinoma	**silent carcinoma**
sychapathic personality		sylkworm gut	**silkworm gut**
	psychopathic personality	symetrical	**symmetrical**
sychiatric	**psychiatric**	symplex	**simplex**
sychoanalysis	**psychoanalysis**	symtomatology	**symptomatology**
sychobioligy	**psychobiology**	symulate	**simulate****
sychodrama	**psychodrama**	synagistic muscle	
sychogenic	**psychogenic**		**synergistic muscle**
sychology	**psychology**	synapptic cleft	**synaptic cleft**
sychonurosis	**psychoneurosis**	syngimy	**syngamy**
sychopathology	**psychopathology**	synis	**sinus****
sychophiseology	**psychophysiology**	synkope	**syncope**

Incorrect	Correct	Incorrect	Correct
synnapsiss	synapsis**	syto- (pre)	cyto-
synoauricular	sinoauricular	sytogenetics	cytogenetics
Syntecks	Syntex	sytollogy	cytology**
synthettic reactions		sytology	cytology**
	synthetic reactions	sytomegalovirus	cytomegalovirus
synusoidal	sinusoidal	sytoplasm	cytoplasm
sysstolic pressure	systolic pressure	sytoscope	cytoscope
syst- (pre)	cyst-	sytosine	cytosine
systemm	system	sytoskeleton	cytoskeleton
systine	cystine	sytoxic T cells	cytotoxic T cells
systitis	cystitis	sytoxin	cytotoxin
systoscopy	cystoscopy	sytte- (pre)	cyt-
syte	site**		

T

Incorrect	Correct	Incorrect	Correct
tabbes dorsalis	tabes dorsalis	tapere	tapir**
tabbetic gate	tabetic gait	tappering	tapering
tabblet	tablet	tapworm	tapeworm
tabel	table	tarrdive dyskinesia	
tabisheer	tabasheer		tardive dyskinesia
tachipnea	tachypnea	tarrget	target
tacksonomy	taxonomy	tarrs/o- (pre)	tars/o-
tacktile	tactile	tarrsus	tarsus
tackycardia	tachycardia	tarsul	tarsal
Tae-Sachs disease		tarter	tartar
	Tay-Sachs disease	tased bud	taste bud
taggatose	tagatose	tash	tache**
tahbso	TAH-BSO	tashes	taches**
tailo- (pre)	talo-	tatoo sergery	tattoo surgery
tainea	taenia**	taurus	torus
taip	tape	taxxonomy	taxonomy
taki- (pre)	tachy-	taylbone	tailbone
tale	tail	tayper	taper**
talebone	tailbone	tayre	tare**
tallipes	talipes	tea-limphocyte	T-lymphocyte
tallis	talus**	teare	tear**
tallose	talose**	tee	tea
tammpon	tampon**	TeeBee	TB
tampann	tampan**	Tee-cell	T cell
tampin	tampon**	teeching hospital	teaching hospital
tampinade	tamponade	teen- (pre)	taen-
Tanea	Taenia**	teeni- (pre)	taeni-
T anned A	T and A	teer	tear** (pron. teer)
tantelem	tantalum	teerduct	tear duct

Incorrect	Correct	Incorrect	Correct
teere	tere**	tere gland	tear gland
teers	tears**	teretology	teratology
teet	teat	teretoma	teratoma
tee-wave	t-wave	tergor	turgor
tegmentle	tegmental	-terigium (suff)	-pterygium
tekneek	technique**	terijeum	pterygium
teknic	technic**	terimicin	Teramycin
teknick	technic**	termenal	terminal
telefase	telephase	TERP	TURP
tell/o/e- (pre)	tel/o/e-	terpentine	turpentine
tella	tela**	terrapsin	terapsin
tellangiectasia	telangiectasia	terrat- (pre)	terat-
temmporal summation		terrato- (pre)	terato-
	temporal summation	terres	teres**
tempel	temple	terrigoid	pterygoid
temperal lobe	temporal lobe	terrin	pterin**
temperel	temporal**	terrminal illness	terminal illness
temperery	temporary	tershiary care	tertiary care
templait	template	tershiary siphilis	tertiary syphilis
tempral	temporal**	tessikal	testicle
tempreture	temperature	tesst- (pre)	test-
tence	tense	tesstis	testis**
tendancy	tendency	tessto- (pre)	testo-
tendemucin	tendomucin	tesstostrone deficiency syndrome ...	
tendenitus	tendinitis**		testosterone deficiency syndrome
tendenus	tendinous**	testical	testicle
tendirness	tenderness**	testikul- (pre)	testicul-
teniss elbow	tennis elbow	testikulo- (pre)	testiculo-
tenn- (pre)	ten-	testiss	testis**
tennaculem	tenaculum	testossterone	testosterone
tenndo- (pre)	tendo-	testube baby	test-tube baby
tenndon	tendon	tetenic convultion ...	
tenned- (pre)	tend-		tetanic convulsion
tennesmus	tenesmus	tetenus	tetanus
tenno- (pre)	teno-	tetenus toxin	tetanus toxin
tennonitis	tenonitis**	teterahidrol cannabinol ...	
tennser	tensor**		tetrahydrocannabinol
tennsure	tensure**	tetiny	tetany
tenshion headaches ...		tetrasicline	tetracycline
	tension headaches	tetrecaine	tetracaine
tentetive diagnosus ...		tettanus	tetanus
	tentative diagnosis	tettra- (pre)	tetra-
tephlon emplant	Teflon implant	thalemic	thalamic
teppid	tepid	thaliddomide	thalidomide
Teramycin	Terramycin	thalisemia	thalassemia
terattogen	teratogen	thallidomide	thalidomide
terbidity	turbidity	thalmus	thalamus
terbinate	turbinate		

Incorrect	Correct
thanatose	thanatos
thannat- (pre)	thanat-
thannato- (pre)	thanato-
thayta	theta
theesis	thesis
theka	theca
thellarche	thelarche
thellitis	thelitis
themometer	thermometer
theraputics	therapeutics
therd	third
therd-degree burn	third-degree burn
therepeutic abortion	therapeutic abortion
therepy	therapy
theretical psychology	theoretical psychology
therippy	therapy
thermajenesis	thermogenesis
therrapeutic window	therapeutic window
therrapist	therapist
therrm- (pre)	therm-
therrmo- (pre)	thermo-
thic filaments	thick filaments
thickning	thickening
thiebone	thighbone
thighroid-stimulating hormone	thyroid-stimulating hormone
thikenned	thickened
thimia (suff)	-thymia
thimin	thymin**
thimine	thiamine**
thimmerosal	thimerosal**
thimus histone	thymus histone
thimyne	thymine**
thinn filaments	thin filaments
thiozanthenes	thioxanthenes
thipental sodium	thiopental sodium
thirmal	thermal
thiroglobulin	thyroglobulin
thiroid	thyroid**
thirotropin	thyrotropin
thiroxin	thyroxin or thyroxine
thiroyd gland	thyroid gland
thisis	phthisis
thorackoplasty	thoracoplasty

Incorrect	Correct
thorassic	thoracic
thoricotomy	thoracotomy
Thorizine	Thorazine
thorrac- (pre)	thorac-
thorracic cavity	thoracic cavity
thorraco- (pre)	thoraco-
thorracostomy	thoracostomy
thorrasi- (pre)	thoraci-
thorrax	thorax
thouracic nerve	thoracic nerve
thracic vertebrae	thoracic vertebrae
threenine	threonine
threshhold	threshold
thretened laber	threatened labor
-thricks (suff)	-thrix
throbing	throbbing
thrombaflebitis	thrombophlebitis
thrombasite	thrombocyte
thrombossis	thrombosis
thrommbine	thrombin
thrommbis	thrombus
thrommboembolism	thromboembolism
throte	throat
thro up	throw up
thruch	thrush
thrumbocytosis	thrombocytosis
thum	thumb
-thurmia (suff)	-thermia
-thurmias (suff)	-thermias
-thurmies (suff)	-thermies
thurmoreceptor	thermoreceptor
-thurmy (suff)	-thermy
thurst	thirst
thy	thigh
thyaridazine	thioridazine
thye	thigh
thyemus	thymus
thyeroid hormone	thyroid hormone
thymen	thymion**
thymole	thymol
thyroyd cartilage	thyroid cartilage
tibamate	tybamate
tibbia	tibia
tibbio- (pre)	tibio-
tibby- (pre)	tibi-
tibeal	tibial

Incorrect	Correct	Incorrect	Correct
tibyal nerve	**tibial nerve**	toebones	**toe bones**
ticc	**tick****	tofaceus goute	**tophaceous gout**
tic dolloreux	**tic douloureux**	tofis	**tophus**
tidde	**tide****	toksemia	**toxemia**
tidil volume	**tidal volume**	toksic shock	**toxic shock**
tieres	**tiers****	toksin	**toxin**
tiflo- (pre)	**typhlo-**	tolarants	**tolerance**
tifus	**typhus**	tolerrence	**tolerance**
tik	**tic****	tollarate	**tolerate**
-tikk (suff)	**-tic**	tollbutanide	**tolbutamide**
Tilenol	**Tylenol**	tollerance	**tolerance**
tilocin	**tylosin**	tollerated	**tolerated**
timpanic membrane		tollnaftate	**tolnaftate**
	tympanic membrane	-tom (suff)	**-tome**
tincter of iodine	**tincture of iodine**	toma- (pre)	**ptoma-**
tinggling	**tingling**	tomain	**ptomaine**
tinia cruris	**tinea cruris**	-tomey (suff)	**-tomy**
tinitus	**tinnitus**	tomoggraphy	**tomography**
tinjed	**tinged**	tonameter	**tonometer**
tinkchure	**tincture**	-tonea (suff)	**-tonia**
Tinnactin	**Tinactin**	-toney (suff)	**-tony**
tinnea	**tinea****	tong	**tongue**
tinnitis	**tinnitis**	tonick	**tonic**
tinya pedis	**tinea pedis**	tonis	**tonus**
tipe	**type**	tonisity	**tonicity**
tipe and cross match		tonngue blade	**tongue blade**
	type and cross match	tonnic	**tonic**
-tiphoid (suff)	**-typhoid**	tonnsil	**tonsil**
tiphoid fever	**typhoid fever**	tonnsilar	**tonsillar**
tipt uterus	**tipped uterus**	tonselectomy	**tonsillectomy**
tirosin	**tyrosine**	tonsil- (pre)	**tonsill-**
tirothricin	**tyrothricin**	tonsilitis	**tonsillitis**
tishew	**tissue**	tonsill and adenoidectomy	
tishue	**tissue**		**tonsil and adenoidectomy**
titanic convulsion		tonsilo- (pre)	**tonsillo-**
	tertanic convulsion	tooba	**tuba****
titejunction	**tight junction**	tooberculin	**tuberculin**
T limphocyte	**T-lymphocyte**	tooberculo- (pre)	**tuberculo-**
toan	**tone**	toobo-insufflation	**tubo-insufflation**
tobercul- (pre)	**tubercul-**	toobo-ovarian pregnancy	
toberosity	**tuberosity**		**tubo-ovarian pregnancy**
tockology	**tocology**	toobo-uterine pregnancy	
tocksic- (pre)	**toxic-**		**tubouterine pregnancy**
tocksico- (pre)	**toxico-**	toobuler	**tubular**
tocksic shock	**toxic shock**	toolaremia	**tularemia**
tocsic shock syndrome		toomer	**tumor**
	toxic shock syndrome	toomor	**tumor**
todeskin	**toad skin**	toonica dartos	**tunica dartos**

tootbrush .... **toothbrush**
tooth-ake .... **toothache**
toothcaping .... **toothcapping**
toothe .... **tooth**
toothpayste .... **toothpaste**
toothpouder .... **toothpowder**
topickal .... **topical**
topp- (pre) .... **top-**
toppo- (pre) .... **topo-**
toreso .... **torso**
tork .... **torque**
torne cartelege .... **torn cartilage**
torper .... torpor
torrpor .... torpor
torsoe .... **torso**
tortion .... **torsion**
tosis .... **ptosis**
tosopherol .... **tocopherol**
-tossis (suff) .... **-ptosis**
totely nonfunctional ....
.... **totally nonfunctional**
tottal mastectomy ....
.... **total mastectomy**
tottic kidney .... **ptotic kidney**
tourista .... **turista**
towe .... **toe****
towell .... towel
tow nail .... **toenail**
toxaplasmosis .... **toxoplasmosis**
toxikosis .... **toxicosis**
toxisity .... **toxicity**
toxx- (pre) .... **tox-**
toxxi- (pre) .... **toxi-**
toxxic .... **toxic**
toxxicology .... **toxicology**
toxxin .... **toxin**
toxxo- (pre) .... **toxo-**
toxxoid .... **toxoid**
trabbeculae .... **trabeculae**
trabeckular .... **trabecular**
trachyotomy .... **tracheotomy****
trackt .... **tracked****
tracktion .... **traction**
tracshon splint .... **traction splint**
traikeal .... **tracheal**
trainning .... **training**
trakea .... **trachea**
trakee- (pre) .... **trache-**

trakeo- (pre) .... **tracheo-**
trakeobronchial ...... **tracheobronchial**
trakt .... **tract****
traktus .... **tractus**
tram .... **TRAM**
tramatic anxiety .... **traumatic anxiety**
trancefusion .... **transfusion**
trancitory .... **transitory**
trangquilyser .... **tranquilizer**
trankwilizer .... **tranquilizer**
trannsfer .... **transfer**
trannsfusion .... **transfusion**
trannsplant .... **transplant**
transducshun .... **transduction**
transdurmal patch ....
.... **transdermal patch**
transduser .... **transducer**
transe .... **trance****
transecshun .... **transection**
transexed .... **transected**
transferin .... **transferrin**
transferrense .... **transference**
transficksion .... **transfixion**
transfrence .... **transference**
transhent situational disorder ....
...... **transient situational disorder**
transishunnal .... **transitional**
translokation .... **translocation**
transmishun .... **transmission**
transpasition .... **transposition****
transporte molecule ....
.... **transport molecule**
transposson .... **transposon****
transvesstism .... **transvestitism**
transvurse colon ...... **transverse colon**
transyurethal resection of the
prostate ....
...... **transurethral resection of the**
prostate
tranz- (pre) ....**trans-****
tranzactional analysis ....
.... **transactional analysis**
trapesius .... **trapezius**
trapezeum .... **trapezium**
trappezoid .... **trapezoid**
trase element .... **trace element**
trasing .... **tracing**
trate .... **trait**

Incorrect	Correct
trawma	trauma
trawma center	trauma center
traycer	tracer
traycheoscopy	tracheoscopy
traycheostomy	tracheostomy
traygus	tragus
trayl	trail**
tredmill	treadmill
treehalose	trehalose
tree mollasses	tree molasses
treepan	trepan
tree shugar	tree sugar
treetment	treatment
trefeen	trephine**
tremer	tremor
tremmor	tremor
tremmulous	tremulous
trennchmouth	trench mouth
trepponema	treponema
triaje	triage
tricanosis	trichinosis
trichoma	trachoma
trick	trich
trick- (pre)	trich-
tricko- (pre)	tricho-
trickomonas	trichomonas
trickomycosis	trichomycosis
tricomonas	trichomonas
tricomycosis	trichomycosis
Tricophyton	Trichophyton
triechomonis vaginalis	*trichomonas vaginalis*
triemesster	trimester
trifluperazine	trifluoperazine
triger	trigger
triggonum	trigonum
triglisserides	triglycerides
trigon	trigone
trijeminal nerve	trigeminal nerve
trikarboxylic acid cycle	tricarboxylic acid cycle
triklormethane	trichloromethane
trikomycosis	trichomycosis
Trinal	Trional
tripanosomiasis	trypanosomiasis
triplette	triplet
tripple	triple
tripsin	trypsin
tripsins	trypsins
trisemy	trisomy
trisepps	triceps
trissiclic compounds	tricyclic compounds
trisyclic antidepressants	tricyclic antidepressants
Trivil	Triavil
Trna	tRNA
troach	troche
trockanter	trochanter
trockiar	trochlear**
trocklear nerve	trochlear nerve
trof- (pre)	troph-
-trofee (suff)	-trophy
troff- (pre)	troph-
-trofic (suff)	-trophic
trofo- (pre)	tropho-
trofoblastic disease	trophoblastic disease
trokar	trocar
trokey	troche
troklea	trochlea**
tromb- (pre)	thromb-
trombo- (pre)	thrombo-
trooth serum	truth serum
tropacal	tropical
-tropea (suff)	-tropia
-trophee (suff)	-trophy
-tropick (suff)	-tropic
troppical medicine	tropical medicine
troppomyosin	tropomyosin
tropponin	troponin
trowma	trauma
truff	trough
trunkus	truncus
trunnk	trunk
tru rib	true rib
trus	truss
try- (pre)	tri-
tryad	triad
tryage	triage
tryal	trial**
tryangular	triangular
tryasylglyceral	triacylglycerol
trybromeothanol	tribromoethanol
tryceps	triceps

trychomonads .... **trichomonads**
trycuspid valve disease ....
.... **tricuspid valve disease**
tryflupromazine .... **triflupromazine**
tryglyceride .... **triglyceride**
tryglycerides .... **triglycerides**
trymester .... **trimester**
tryppsins .... **trypsins**
tryptafan .... **tryptophan**
Tsanck test .... **Tzanck test**
tubbal ligation .... **tubal ligation**
tubbercul- (pre)................... **tubercul-**
tubbus .... **tubus****
tubektomy .... **tubectomy**
tubel .... **tubal****
tubercullo- (pre)................. **tuberculo-**
tubercyulin test .... **tuberculin test**
tuberrcullosis .... **tuberculosis**
tubil insufflation .... **tubal insufflation**
tuble pregnancy .... **tubal pregnancy**
tubor.............................. **tuber****
tubrosity .... **tuberosity**
tuburcle .... **tubercle**
tubz .... **tubes****
tuch .... **touch**
Tuenal .... **Tuinal**
tullaremia .... **tularemia**
tumer.................................. **tumor**
tumessence .... **tumescence**
trumessent .... **tumescent**
Tumms .... **Tums**
tungue depressor.... **tongue depressor**
tunika albuginea ..... **tunica albuginea**

tunnle .... **tunnel**
Turette's syndrome ....
.... **Tourette's syndrome**
turm..**term**
turminal .... **terminal**
turniquet .... **tourniquet**
tusis .... **tussis**
tutch .... **touch**
tuth bonding .... **tooth bonding**
twich .... **twitch**
twilite ....**twilight**
twobo-insufflation ....
.... **tubo-insufflation**
twobo-ovarian pregnancy ....
.... **tubo-ovarian pregnancy**
twobo-uterine pregnancy ....
.... **tubouterine pregnancy**
twylight ....**twilight**
tybeofibuler .... **tibiofibular**
tybia .... **tibia**
tyde .... **tied****
tyfoid................................**typhoid**
tylin ....**ptyalin**
Tylinal ....**Tylenol**
typhis fever .... **typhus fever**
Tyrpanosoma gambiense ....
.... **Trypanosoma gambiense**
-tysis (suff) ....**-ptysis**
tyter....................................... **titer**
tyubal .... **tubal****
tyube .... **tube**
tyunica .... **tunica**

U

ubradant .... **abradant**
ubrasion ....**abrasion**
ubsessive-compulsive neurosis ....
..... **obsessive-compulsive neurosis**
ucalyptus ....**eucalyptus**
ukaryote ....**eukaryote**
ulcerrative colitis ..... **ulcerative colitis**
ulectroforeesis........... **electrophoresis**
ulln/o- (pre) .... **uln/o-**
ullner................................... **ulnar****

ullserate .... **ulcerate**
ulltera- (pre)............................... **ultra-**
ulltrafiltrate ....**ultrafiltrate**
ulne .... **ulna****
ulner nerve ....**ulnar nerve**
ulser .... **ulcer**
ulterasound .... **ultrasound**
ultersonic therapy ....
.... **ultrasonic therapy**
ultersonography ...... **ultrasonography**

Incorrect	Correct	Incorrect	Correct

ultravilet therapy .... ultraviolet therapy
umbilickus .... umbilicus
umbillical .... umbilical
umergency ward ..... emergency ward
unaversal antidote..........................
.... universal antidote
unbilical cord .... umbilical cord
uncommpensated care ....
.... uncompensated care
unconnscious .... unconscious
unconsshous.................... unconscious
uncontrolible .... uncontrollable
undabite .... underbite
undecended .... undescended
underrarm .... underarm
underwait .... underweight
undetermined .... undetermined
undiferentiated .... undifferentiated
undyulent fever.......... undulent fever
uneekly abled .... uniquely abled
unekwivical diagnosis ....
.... unequivocal diagnosis
unesthetist .... anesthetist
ungwal .... ungual**
ungwent .... unguent
ungyula .... ungula**
unichoidism .... eunuchoidism
unik .... eunuch**
unnconventinal slow virus
infections ....
.... unconventional slow virus
infections
unnilaterel .... unilateral
unnown .... unknown
unofishill .... unofficial
unsatchurated fat ...... unsaturated fat
unstabel .... unstable
unvacsinated .... unvaccinated
uper arm .... upper arm
Upjon .... Upjohn
uppa respiratory infection ....
.... upper respiratory infection
uppar GI series .... upper GI series
uppra extremities ....
.... upper extremities
uralania .... urolagnia

uralogy .... urology
uranalysis .... urinalysis
urathritis......................... urethritis
ureater .... ureter**
ureemia vesicle .... uremia vesicle
ureeter- (pre)........................... ureter-
ureetero- (pre)..................... uretero-
ureethr- (pre) .... urethr-
ureethra .... urethra**
ureethro- (pre) .... urethro-
uremmic .... uremic
uria .... urea
uricil...................................... uracil
urick acid .... uric acid
urin...................................... urine
urinary track .... urinary tract
urinery bladder .... urinary bladder
urinil .... uranyl**
urinnale .... urinal**
urinnary tract infection..................
.... urinary tract infection
urinnation .... urination
urinne .... urine
urophollitropin .... urofollitropin
urowlogical .... urological
urranal .... urinal**
urrano- (pre) .... urono-
-urrea (suff) .... -uria
urric acid .... uric acid
urrinary .... urinary
urrun- (pre) .... urin-
urruno- (pre) .... urino-
urtacaria .... urticaria
urthane .... urethane
US reccomended daily allowance...
.... U.S. recommended daily
allowance
utarine contractions ....
.... uterine contractions
uterous .... uterus
uterrus .... uterus
utherly abled .... otherly abled
utillization review committee ....
.... utilization review committee
utiri .... uteri
utterine contractant ....
.... uterine contractant

100

Incorrect	Correct
uttricle	**utricle**
utur- (pre)	**uter-**
uturo- (pre)	**utero-**
uvial	**uveal****
uvulay	**uvulae**
uvvula	**uvula****
uvyularr	**uvular****

V

Incorrect	Correct
vacceen	**vaccine****
vacsine therapy	**vaccine therapy**
vacume	**vacuum**
vacume aspiration	**vacuum aspiration**
vaganal cream	**vaginal cream**
vagenitis	**vaginitis**
vagg- (pre)	**vag-**
vaggel	**vagal**
vaggin/i- (pre)	**vagin/i-**
vaggo- (pre)	**vago-**
vaginizmus	**vaginismus**
vaginnal foam	**vaginal foam**
VA hosspital	**VA hospital**
vaig	**vague**
vaine	**vein**
vajina	**vagina**
vajino- (pre)	**vagino-**
vajinolabial	**vagionolabial**
vajinorectal	**vaginorectal**
vakcination	**vaccination**
vaksin	**vaccin**
vakuole	**vacuole**
vallerian	**valerian**
vallgis	**valgus**
valline	**valine**
Vallium	**Valium****
vallt	**vault**
vallve	**valve****
vallvula	**valvula****
Valsaver maneuver	**Valsalva's maneuver**
valum	**vallum****
valveotomy	**valvotomy**
valver	**valva****
valviewlotomy	**valvulotomy**
valvuel/o- (pre)	**valvul/o-**
valvulay	**valvulae****

Incorrect	Correct
valvyalar heart disease	**valvular heart disease**
valvyeler	**valvular****
vanncomycin	**vancomycin**
vaperise	**vaporize**
vapers	**vapors**
varacose veins	**varicose veins**
varecose	**varicose**
varicks	**varix**
varikoseal	**varicocele**
varisella	**varicella**
varric/o- (pre)	**varic/o-**
varricosity	**varicosity**
varriola	**variola**
varrus	**varus**
varycose vanes	**varicose veins**
vasadillation	**vasodilation**
vasektemy	**vasectomy**
vasel	**vasal****
vasidilator	**vasodilator**
vaskular system	**vascular system**
vasoecongestion	**vasocongestion**
vasscularity	**vascularity**
vasscular spiders	**vascular spiders**
vass diferens	**vas deferens**
vassectomy	**vasectomy**
vassed	**vast****
vasso- (pre)	**vaso-**
vassoconstrictor	**vasoconstrictor**
vassometer	**vasometer**
vassopressin	**vasopressin**
vaygus nerve	**vagus nerve**
-vaylent (suff)	**-valent**
vaz	**vas****
vaz/o- (pre)	**vas/o-**
vazcul/o- (pre)	**vascul/o-**
Vazeline	**Vaseline**
vazoconstriction	**vasoconstriction**

vazopressor .... **vasopressor**
vd .... **VD**
vee-dee .... **VD**
veena cava .... **vena cava**
veenous .... **venous****
veenous thrombosis ....
.... **venous thrombosis**
vegtable albumin ....
.... **vegetable albumin**
veigal .... **vagal**
veilence .... **valence**
-veillence (suff) .... -**valence**
vejetative state .... **vegetative state**
vektor .... **vector****
-velemia (suff) .... -**volemia**
vellpo .... **Velpeau**
vellum .... **velum**
venagraphy .... **venography**
veneerial .... **venereal**
vener caver .... **vena cava**
venil- (pre) .... **venul-**
venilo- (pre) .... **venulo-**
venireal disease .... **venereal disease**
-venis (suff) .... -**venous**
venna .... **vena****
venni- (pre) .... **veni-**
venno- (pre) .... **veno-**
venntral .... **ventral**
venntricular fibrillation ....
.... **ventricular fibrillation**
vennule .... **venule****
vennus .... **venus****
ventelation .... **ventilation**
venter/i/o- (pre) .... **ventr/i/o-**
venterculography ... **ventriculography**
-ventrel (suff) .... -**ventral**
ventrickal .... **ventricle**
ventrickuler .... **ventricular**
venus .... **venous****
venus disorders .... **venous disorders**
venypuncture .... **venipuncture**
venyula .... **venula**
venelar .... **venular****
vergin .... **virgin**
veriform appendix ....
.... **vermiform appendix**
verjens .... **vergence****
vermickuler .... **vermicular**

vermiside .... **vermicide**
vershun .... **version**
vertabray .... **vertebrae**
vertecal .... **vertical****
vertecks .... **vertex****
vertegoe .... **vertigo**
vertibra .... **vertebra**
verrtebral column ....
.... **vertebral column**
vertickle .... **verticil****
veruca .... **verruca**
vesecal .... **vesical****
vesicala .... **vesicular****
vesiccul/o- (pre) .... **vesicul/o-**
vesickula .... **vesicula****
vessell .... **vessel****
vessica .... **vesica****
vessicle .... **vesicle****
vessico- (pre) .... **vesico-**
vesstibular nerve ...... **vestibular nerve**
vestebule .... **vestibule**
vestibbulitis .... **vestibulitis**
vestibuller system ....
.... **vestibular system**
vestijal organ .... **vestigial organ**
vetarinary medicine ....
.... **veterinary medicine**
vetran's hospital ... **veteran's hospital**
vetrinarian .... **veterinarian**
vetterinary .... **veterinary**
vibbrio .... **vibrio****
Vibreo .... *Vibrio***
vibritory sensation ....
.... **vibratory sensation**
vicid .... **viscid**
victimmization .... **victimization**
vidiyan .... **vidian**
viecarious .... **vicarious**
vierus .... **virus****
vigerous exersise ... **vigorous exercise**
vilis .... **villus****
vilose .... **villose****
vilous .... **villous** or **villose****
vin/i/o- (pre) .... **ven/i/o-**
vinae .... **venae****
Vinsent angina .... **Vincent's angina**
virall infection .... **viral infection**
viril diseases .... **viral diseases**

Incorrect	Correct
virilizing	**viralizing**
virjense	**vergence****
virlization	**virilization**
virrile	**virile****
virrology	**virology**
viryulent	**virulent**
visid	**viscid**
viskis	**viscus****
viskous	**viscous****
vissera	**viscera**
visseral	**visceral**
vissid	**viscid**
vitaline	**vitelline****
vitammin deficiency	**vitamin deficiency**
vitil	**vital**
vitil capacity	**vital capacity**
vitimin	**vitamin**
vitrious humor	**vitreous humor**
vittellin	**vitellin****
vittro	**vitro**
Vixx Vaporub	**Vicks Vaporub**
vize	**vise****
vizible	**visible**
vizon	**vision**
vizual	**visual**
vocall fold	**vocal fold**
vocks	**vox**
voela	**vola****
voise box	**voice box**
vokal cords	**vocal cords**
volcella	**volsella**
voler arches	**volar arches**
volintary muscle	**voluntary muscle**
voller	**volar****
volletile	**volatile**
vollitional	**volitional**

Incorrect	Correct
volluntary nervous system	**voluntary nervous system**
-vollute (suff)	**-volute**
volv- (pre)	**vulv-**
volvitis	**vulvitis**
volvo- (pre)	**vulvo-**
volyume	**volume**
vommer	**vomer**
vommiting	**vomiting**
-vorrus (suff)	**-vorous**
vorteks	**vortex****
voyd	**void**
vue	**view**
vueing instrument	**viewing instrument**
vullgaris	**vulgaris**
vullva	**vulva****
vulseller	**vulsella**
vulver	**vulvar****
vulver distrophy	**vulvar dystrophy**
vurgins	**virgins****
vurmi- (pre)	**vermi-**
vurmifuge	**vermifuge**
vurtibr- (pre)	**vertebr-**
vurtibro- (pre)	**vertebro-**
vurtigo	**vertigo**
vwyurism	**voyeurism**
vyable	**viable**
vyce	**vice****
vynil	**vinyl**
vyomicin	**viomycin**
vyral	**viral****
vyroid	**viroid**
vyrus	**virus****
vyta- (pre)	**vita-**
vytal signs	**vital signs**
vytamin	**vitamin**

W

Incorrect	Correct
wacks-like secretion	**wax-like secretion**
wahrt	**wart**
waight	**weight****
waisste	**waist****
waisting	**wasting**

Incorrect	Correct
wait bearing	**weight bearing**
waker	**walker**
waksy flexibility	**waxy flexibility**
waleye	**walleye**
wandring pacemaker	**wandering pacemaker**

warred	**ward****	white sell	**white cell**
warrfarin	**warfarin**	white wacks	**white wax**
Warrner Chilcot	**Warner Chilcott**	whoo	**WHO**
wartt	**wart****	whume	**womb**
Wassiman test	**Wassermann test**	whydening	**widening**
wate	**wait****	whydspread	**widespread**
wate bareing	**weight bearing**	why-shaped scar	**Y-shaped scar**
wating room	**waiting room**	why-type incision	**Y-type incision**
wattery eyes	**watery eyes**	wich hazel	**witch hazel**
Wattson	**Watson**	winpipe	**windpipe**
wayst	**waist****	wiplash	**whiplash**
webb spase	**web space**	wiplash injery	**whiplash injury**
weekness	**weakness**	wite blood cell	**white blood cell**
weel	**wheal****	wites	**whites**
weelchair	**wheelchair**	withdrall reflex	**withdrawal reflex**
weening	**weaning**	with drawal simptoms	
weesand	**weasand**		**withdrawal symptoms**
weezing	**wheezing**	withdrawen	**withdrawn**
weighting room	**waiting room**	withdrawl	**withdrawal**
wej recection	**wedge resection**	with-in	**within**
well baby care	**well-baby care**	withring	**withering**
well healed scar	**well-healed scar**	witlow	**whitlow**
wellt	**welt**	wizdom tooth	**wisdom tooth**
wel-woman clinic		Wolfian body	**Wolffian body**
	well-woman clinic	woom	**womb**
wenn	**wen****	woomb	**womb**
weppon	**weapon**	woond	**wound**
werk up	**work-up**	worl	**whorl**
werkup	**work-up**	worled sells	**whorled cells**
World Health Organization		would sugar	**wood sugar**
	World Health Organization	wrasp	**rasp**
werlpool bath	**whirlpool bath**	wrestlessness	**restlessness**
werm	**worm**	wrest pain	**rest pain**
Westrin blot	**Western blot**	wright atrium	**right atrium**
wey	**whey****	wrisst	**wrist**
weyy	**way****	wryeneck	**wryneck**
wharfarin	**warfarin**	wume	**womb**
whart	**wart****	wunder drug	**wonder drug**
whele	**wheel****	wurd salad	**word salad**
whelt	**welt**	wurk up	**work-up**
which hasel	**witch hazel**	wurms	**worms**
whick	**wick**	wyde local incision	
whipplash	**whiplash**		**wide local incision**
white hed	**whitehead**	Wyith-Ayerst	**Wyeth-Ayerst**
whiteish placks	**whitish plaques**		

X

Incorrect	Correct	Incorrect	Correct
xant- (pre)	**xanth-**	x-rae	**x-ray**
Xantac	**Zantac**	xraye therapy	**x-ray therapy**
xanto- (pre)	**xantho-**	xray teknician	**x-ray technician**
x kromosome	**x-chromosome**		

Y

Incorrect	Correct	Incorrect	Correct
yawse	**yaws**	yuran- (pre)	**uran-**
yeest	**yeast**	yurano- (pre)	**urano-**
yelow fever	**yellow fever**	yurea	**urea**
yelowish discharge	**yellowish discharge**	yuremia	**uremia**
yelow marow	**yellow marrow**	yuremic	**uremic**
y kromosome	**y-chromosome**	yuretal	**uretal**
yoke sac	**yolk sac**	yurethr- (pre)	**urethr-**
yoke stalk	**yolk stalk**	yurethra	**urethra****
yores	**yaws**	yurethral	**urethral**
youni- (pre)	**uni-**	yurethro- (pre)	**urethro-**
your- (pre)	**ur-**	yuretic ridge	**uretic ridge**
-yourea (suff)	**-urea**	yuric- (pre)	**uric-**
youreter	**ureter****	yurico- (pre)	**urico-**
-youria (suff)	**-uria**	yurination	**urination**
youro- (pre)	**uro-**	yurine	**urine**
yourology	**urology**	yuro- (pre)	**uro-**
yourrea	**urea**	yurogenital	**urogenital**
youstachian tube	**eustachian tube**	yurological	**urological**
youvia	**uvea****	yuroscopy	**uroscopy**
you wave	**U wave**	yuter- (pre)	**uter-**
youze	**use**	yuteria	**uteri**
-yular (suff)	**-ular**	yuterine	**uterine**
-yulem (suff)	**-ulum**	yutero- (pre)	**utero-**
-yulent (suff)	**-ulent**	yutero-ovarian varicosele	**utero-ovarian vericocele**
yulo- (pre)	**ulo-**	yuteropelvic junction	**uteropelvic junction**
-yulus (suff)	**-ulus**	yuterus	**uterus**
Yung	**Jung**	yuthanasia	**euthanasia**
yuni- (pre)	**uni-**	yuvitis	**uveitis**
yuppy flu	**yuppie flue**		
yur- (pre)	**ur-**		

Z

Incorrect	Correct
zanax	**xanax**
zanth- (pre)	**xanth-**
zantheen	**xanthene****
zanthin	**xanthine****
zantho- (pre)	**xantho-**
zanthochromatic fluid	**xanthochromatic fluid**
zanthoma	**xanthoma**
zee-flap	**Z-flap**
zeero	**zero****
zeno- (pre)	**xeno-**
zer- (pre)	**xer-**
zero- (pre)	**xero-****
zerosis	**xerosis**
zerostomia	**xerostoma**
zerro- (pre)	**xero-****
zew- (pre)	**zoo-**
Ziess	**Zeiss**
zifft	**ZIFT** or **Zift**
ziffy- (pre)	**xiphi-**
zifo- (pre)	**xipho-**
zifoid process	**xiphoid process**
ziglo- (pre)	**zyglo-**
zigoma	**zygoma**
zigomatic	**zygomatic**
zigomatic arch	**zygomatic arch**
zigomaticofacial nerve	**zygomaticofacial nerve**
zigomatic reflex	**zygomatic reflex**

Incorrect	Correct
zilo- (pre)	**xylo-**
zime- (pre)	**zyme-**
-zimme (suff)	**-zyme**
zimo- (pre)	**zymo-**
zimogen granule	**zymogen granule**
zinck oxide	**zinc oxide**
zinc oyntment	**zinc ointment**
zine	**zein**
zink	**zinc**
ziph/i/o- (pre)	**xiph/i/o-**
zoan	**zone**
Zoevirax	**Zovirax**
zonosis	**zoonosis**
zonullar cataract	**zonular cataract**
zonulle fibres	**zonule fibers**
-zooic (suff)	**-zoic**
zosster	**zoster**
zow- (pre)	**zo-**
-zune (suff)	**-zoon**
-zyote (suff)	**-zoite**
zweiback	**zwieback**
zyfee- (pre)	**xiphi-**
zygoat intra-fallopian transfer	**zygote intra-fallopian transfer**
zygot	**zygote**
zylo- (pre)	**xylo-**
zylose	**xylose**
zypho- (pre)	**xipho-**
zyster	**xyster**

Words Commonly Confused Because They Look Alike or Sound Alike

A

abductor (part-separating muscle) •
adductor (that which pulls muscle
to median)

ablatio (detached retina) • ablation
(tissue removal)

ablation—see ablatio

abortin (glycerin extract) • abortion
(termination of pregnancy)

abortion—see abortin

absorb (to take in) • adsorb (to hold
on surface)

Acacia—see acacia

acacia (emolient in medicines) •
Acacia (tree yielding medicinal
herbs)

acapnia (low carbon dioxide) •
acapnial (with low carbon
dioxide)

acapnial—see acapnia

acarid (a mite) • acid (sour; water-
soluble compound) • acrid
(corrosive, bitter)

acathexia (unable to retain
secretions) • acathexis (mental
disorder)

acathexis—see acathexia

acetal (clear liquid) • acetyl (acetic
acid molecule)

acetyl—see acetal

acid—see acarid

acorea (lacking eye pupil) • acoria
(not satiated)

acoria—see acorea

acrid—see acarid

additive (substance added to a basic
food or chemical) • auditive (able
to learn more by hearing)

adductor—see abductor

adsorb—see absorb

aerocele (distention with gas) •
aerosol (fine mist)

aerogenous (gas-forming) •
erogenous (causing sexual
arousal)

aerosol—see aerocele

affect (major emotion; to cause) •
effect (a result; to bring about)

afferent (toward a central organ) •
efferent (centrifugal)

affluent (freely flowing) • effluent
(flowing outward)

agar (seaweed extract) • agger
(projection)

agger—see agar

aides (assistants; helpers) • aids
(helps; assists) • AIDS (acquired
immune deficiency syndrome)

aids—see aides

AIDS—see aides

ailment (illness) • aliment (food)

alangine (alkaloid emetic) • alanine
(a natural amino acid) • Al-Anon
(Alcoholics Anonymous) • alantin
(diagnostic agent for kidney tests)

alanine—see alangine

Al-Anon—see alangine

alantin—see alangine

albumen (egg white) • albumin
(water-soluble protein) • albumin-
(prefix for water-soluble protein
compounds)

albumin—see albumen

albumin-—see albumen

aliment—*see* ailment

alimentary (canal for digesting food) • elementary (simple; basic)

Allergan (maker of eye products) • allergen (allergy-causing antigen)

allergen—*see* Allergan

allopath (practitioner of allopathy) • allopathy (system of cure by creating antagonistic symptoms)

allopathy—*see* allopath

allotrophic (made nonnutritious) • allotropic (concerned about others; showing more forms)

allotropic—*see* allotrophic

ameleia (apathy) • amelia (congenital loss of limbs)

amelia—*see* ameleia

amidin (soluble starch) • amidine (a radical)

amidine—*see* amidin

aminopurine (part of DNA and RNA) • aminopyrine (an analgesic)

aminopyrine—*see* aminopurine

amorphous (shapeless) • amorphus (malformed fetus)

amorphus—*see* amorphous

ampul or ampule (small container) • ampulla (tubular dilatation)

ampulla—*see* ampul or ampule

anaclasis (refraction) • anaclisis (state of reclining)

anaclisis—*see* anaclasis

anal (pertaining to the anus; psychological stage) • anol (carcinogenic compound)

analyses—*see* analysis

analysis (identification of ingredients; psychoanalysis) • analyses (pl. of *analysis*) • analyzes (breaks down problems into parts)

analyzes—*see* analysis

androgenous (creating male offspring) • androgynous (with male and female characteristics)

androgynous—*see* androgenous

anger (wrath) • angor (distress)

angiohypertonia (vessel constriction) • angiohypotonia (vessel dilation)

angiohypotonia—*see* angiohypertonia

angor—*see* anger

anima (one's inner self) • animal (sentient being) • enema (cleansing)

animal—*see* anima

animus (hatred) • anomous (lacking shoulders)

anise (seed that relieves gas) • anus (rectal opening) • heinus (evil)

annulose (ring-like) • annulus or anulus (ring)

annulus or anulus—*see* annulose

anol—*see* anal

anomia (inability to name objects) • anomie (disorientation, isolation)

anomie—*see* anomia

anomous—*see* animus

anorchous (lacking testes) • anorchus (one without testes)

anorchus—*see* anorchus

ante- (prefix for *before*) • anti- (prefix for *against*)

antedate (to precede; to fix at an earlier date) • antidote (a poison remedy) anti-—*see* ante-

antidote—*see* antedate

antimer (mirror-image molecule) •
antimere (symmetrical; right
angled)

antimere—*see* antimer

anulus—*see* annulose

anus—*see* anise

apatite (mineral group) • appetite
(desire)

aphagia (inability to swallow) •
aphakia (lacking crystalline lens)
• aphasia (loss or weakening of
linguistic ability)

aphakia—*see* aphagia

aphasia—*see* aphagia

aphrodisia (state of sexual arousal) •
aphrodisiac (a sexual stimulant)

aphrodisiac—*see* aphrodisia

appetite—*see* apatite

araban (pectin constituent) • arabin
(gum)

arabin—*see* araban

arhythmia or arrhythmia (irregular
heart beat) • erythema (abnormal
skin flushing)

arrythmia—*see* arythmia

arteritis (arterial inflammation) •
arthritis (inflammation of joints)

arthritis—*see* arteritis

asbestos (fibrous material causing
lung disease) • asbestosis (lung
disease)

asbestosis—*see* asbestos

atomic (pertaining to the atom) •
atonic (lacking normal strength)

atonic—*see* atomic

auditive—*see* additive

aura (pre-epilectic feeling) • aural
(of the ear) • oral (relating to the
mouth; spoken)

aural—*see* aura

automatin (bovine extract) •
automation (self-acting
mechanisms) • automaton (robot)

automation—*see* automatin

automaton—*see* automatin

auxiliary—*see* axillary

avoid (to prevent from happening) •
ovoid (egg-shaped)

axillary (relating to the armpit) •
auxiliary (helping; subsidiary)

axiom (accepted truth) • axion (spinal
cord and brain) • axon or axone
(the body's axis) • exon (an
interrupted gene)

axion—*see* axiom

axogenous (stemming from an axion)
• exogenous (stemming from
external causes)

axon—*see* axiom

axone—*see* axiom

B

Bachman (test for trichinosis) •
Bachmann (band of muscle
fibers)

Bachmann—*see* Bachman

bacilli (microorganisms) • bacillin
(antibiotic)

bacillin—*see* bacilli

bactericide (bacteria-killing agent) •

bacteriocidin (antibacterial antibody) • **bacteriocin** (antibacterial bacteria)

bacteriocidin—*see* bactericide

bacteriocin—*see* bactericide

bacteriophage (a virus) • **bacteriophagia** (destruction of bacteria)

bacteriophagia—*see* bacteriophage

bacteriotropic (changing bacteria) • **bacteriotropin** (immune serum component)

bacteriotropin—*see* bacteriotropic

bacteroid (like bacteria; modified bacteria) • ***Bacteroides*** (bacteria found in mouth or bowel)

Bacteroides—*see* bacteroid

Baelz (labial inflammation) • **Bayle's** (paralysis of the insane)

Baer (method for adhesions) • **Baeyer** (test for dextrose)

Baeyer—*see* Baer

balance (equilibrium; weighing instrument) • **Ballance** (sign in splenic rupture)

bald (without hair) • **ball** (round mass) • **bawl** (to cry)

ball—*see* bald

Ballance—*see* balance

balm (soothing ointment) • **Balme** (cough when prone)

Balme—*see* balm

bar (upper gums of a horse) • **Bar** (incision of a cesarean section)

Bar—*see* bar

basal (at or near the base) • **basil** (aromatic plant)

based (served as base) • **bast** (fiber used in surgery)

bases (pl. of *basis*) • **basis** (base of a structure)

basil—*see* basal

basis—*see* bases

bast—*see* based

bath (immersal for cleaning) • **bathe** (to take a bath or swim)

bathe—*see* bath

bawl—*see* bald

Bayle's—*see* Baelz

bel (acoustic ratio) • **Bell** (physiologist; palsy specialist)

belie (to contradict; to show as false) • **belly** (stomach)

Bell—*see* bel

belly—*see* belie

benzene (coal tar by-product; dissolves sulfur) • **benzin** or **benzine** (oil by-product; solvent in compounds) • **benzoin** (balsamic resin)

benzin—*see* benzene

benzine—*see* benzene

benzoin—*see* benzene

benzoyl (benzoic acid radical) • **benzyl** (hydrocarbon radical)

benzyl—*see* benzoyl

berth (bed; job) • **birth** (the bringing into life)

beta (the Greek letter that distinguishes isomers) • ***Beta*** (plant genus, e.g., beets) • **better** (improved, healthy)

Beta—*see* beta

better—*see* beta

Bial (reagent) • bile (liver secretion)

bias (angle; systemic error) • bios (single-cell organism's growth factor) • biose (sugar with two carbon atoms) • biosis (vitality)

bile—*see* Bial

bios—*see* bias

biose—*see* bias

biosis—*see* bias

biotech (short for *biotechnology*) • biotic (pertaining to life)

biotic—*see* biotech

birth—*see* berth

bisulfate (an acid sulfate) • bisulfide (disulfide) • bisulfite (acid sulfite)

bilsulfide—*see* bisulfate

bisulfite—*see* bisulfate

blackout (a fainting spell) • black out (to faint)

black out—*see* blackout

bloc (a group working together) • Bloch (biochemist, Nobel Prize winner) • block (an obstruction; to obstruct) • Blocq (French physician; Blocq's disease)

Bloch—*see* bloc

block—*see* bloc

Blocq—*see* bloc

born (came to life) • borne (carried)

borne—*see* born

bowel (intestine) • bowl (a basin)

bowl—*see* bowel

bradyphagia (abnormal slowness in eating) • bradyphasia (abnormal slowness in speaking)

bradyphasia—*see* bradyphagia

brake (to slow; to halt) • break (to cause a rupture)

breach (to break or violate) • breech (buttocks)

breadth (width) • breath (drawing air into and expelling air from the lungs) • breathe (to take a breath)

break—*see* brake

breakout (sudden eruption) • break out (to get a skin eruption)

break out—*see* breakout

breath—*see* breadth

breathe—*see* breadth

breech—*see* breach

bright (radiating light) • Bright (physician whose work is associated with study of blindness)

Bright—*see* bright

bronchial (pertaining to bronchi) • bronchiole (bronchial subdivision without cartilage)

bronchiole—*see* bronchial

buba (tropical disease— leishmaniasis) • bubo (lymph node inflammation)

bubo—*see* buba

bud (small part of an embryo) • Budd (jaundice specialist)

Budd—*see* bud

bulbous (like a bulb) • bulbus (enlarged mass)

bulbus—*see* bulbous

buts (refusals, delays) • butts (makes two objects come into contact)

butts—*see* buts

C

calcine (to reduce to a dry powder using heat) • calicine (like a calix)

calculous (pertaining to multiple stones) • calculus (hard mass) • caliculus (cup-shaped body)

calculus—see calculous

calicine—see calcine

caliculus—see calculous

calix or calyx (cup-shaped organ) • calx (the heel; chalk)

call (request; summons; phone) • caul (birth amnion)

callose (bean extract polysaccharide) • callous (hard; unemotional) • callus (thick skin)

callous—see callose

callus—see callose

calor (heat) • collar (band, usually on neck) • color (hue, lightness)

calx—see calix

calyx—see calix

camphor (oil for flatulence) • chamfer (a groove)

cancer (a malignant tumor) • canker (lip or mouth ulcer) • chancre (ulceration; symptom of serious disease)

Candida (organism that produces a yeastlike infection) • candidid (skin eruption)

candidid—see Candida

canker—see cancer

cannabism (morbid state from marijuana use) • cannibalism (one cell eating another)

cannibalism—see cannabism

capelet (horse's swelling) • caplet (enclosed medication)

capita (pl. of caput—head of the body) • capital (of the femur's head)

capital—see capita

capitation (fee for medical care) • captation (first stage of hypnotism)

caplet—see capelet

caproin (glycerin caproate) • caprone (volatile oil)

caprone—see caproin

capsula (fibrous envelopment) • capsule (medical dose container)

capsule—see capsula

captation—see capitation

carate (skin disease) • carrot (edible root)

carbuncle (boil) • caruncle (fleshy swelling)

-cardia (suffix for part of the stomach) • cardiac (relating to the heart)

cardiac—see -cardia

cardioid (like the heart) • carotid (main neck artery)

career (job; chance for advancement) • carer (one who takes care of or assists) • carrier (transmitter of disease)

carer—see career

caries (tooth or bone decay) • carries (harbors, transports)

carotid—see cardioid

carrier—see career

carries—see caries

carrot—*see* carate

caruncle—*see* carbuncle

cataphora (extreme lethargy) • cataphoria (vision disorder)

cataphoria—*see* cataphora

cauda (tail-like appendage) • cauter (tissue-destroying heating instrument)

caul—*see* call

cauter—*see* cauda

cava (a main vein) • cave (enclosed cavity)

cave—*see* cava

-cele (suffix indicating *swelling*) • cell (minute mass) • seal (firm closure)

cell—*see* -cele

censor (psychic influence; ban) • sensor (measuring device)

census (a counting; characteristics of a group) • senses (faculties of sight, hearing, touch, etc.)

cerated (covered with wax or fat) • serrated (with sawlike edges)

cereal (edible grain) • serial (occurring in a series)

cerebellum (the lower part of the brain) • cerebrum (the front and largest part of the brain)

cerebrum—*see* cerebellum

cereous (waxlike) • Cereus (type of cactus) • cerous (relating to rare metals) • serious (grave)

Cereus—*see* cereous

cerous—*see* cereous

cerumen (waxy ear secretion) • serum (immune blood injection)

chalasia (relaxation of sphincter) • chalaza (albuminous band)

chalaza—*see* chalasia

chamfer—*see* camphor

chancre—*see* cancer

chart (patient's record) • charta (medicated paper)

charta—*see* chart

chlorophenol (antiseptic) • chlorphenol (acid-base indicator)

chlorphenol—*see* chlorophenol

cholecystis (gall bladder) • cholecystitis (inflammation of gall bladder)

cholecystitis—*see* cholecystis

choleraic (related to cholera) • choleric (enraged)

choleric—*see* choleraic

cilium (eyelids or their hair) • psyllium (plantago seed)

cine (combining form referring to movement) • sign (indication)

cirrus (flexible animal appendage) • scirrhous (relating to carcinoma) • scirrhus (a carcinoma) • serous (relating to serum)

cite (to use as an example) • -cyte (suffix indicating *type of cell*) • sight (vision) • site (location)

coccus (round bacterium) • *Coccus* (insects used in biological stain)

Coccus—*see* coccus

cochlea (bone cavity) • cochlear (of the bone cavity) • cochleare (spoon or spoonful)

cochlear—*see* cochlea

cochleare—*see* cochlea

colds (viral inflammations) • coles (penis or clitoris) • Colles (surgeon) coles—*see* colds

collar—*see* calor

Colles—*see* colds

collum (neck) • column (pillar-like structure)

color—*see* calor

column—*see* collum

compact (packed closely) • compacta (dense portion of uterus lining)

compacta—*see* compact

complement (to make complete) • compliment (to praise)

compliment—*see* complement

conscience (sense of right and wrong) • conscious (aware; awake)

conscious—*see* conscience

contact (touching; a disease carrier) • contract (formal agreement)

contract—*see* contact

cor (heart) • core (central part)

core—*see* cor

coronary (related to the heart) • coroner (medical examiner)

coroner—*see* coronary

corpse (dead body) • corpus (body)

corpus—*see* corpse

creatine (muscle extractive) • creatinine (urine component)

creatinine—*see* creatine

crus (leg; a leglike part) • crust (hard outer layer)

crust—*see* crus

crystallin (globulin in eye lens) • crystalline (transparent)

crystalline—*see* crystallin

-cyte—*see* cite

cytology (study of cell structure) • sitology (dietetics)

D

daily (every day) • dally (to waste time)

dally—*see* daily

days (pl. of *day*—24 hours) • daze (bewildered)

daze—*see* days

dead (not living) • deed (act; a legal document)

decade (ten years) • decayed (rotted; fell apart)

decayed—*see* decade

decadent (having low moral standards) • decedent (a dead person)

decease (to die) • disease (sick)

decedent—*see* decadent

decent (good; honest) • descent (downward movement)

dechloridation (reducing the amount of chlorine) • dechlorination (removing all chlorine)

dechlorination—*see* dechloridation

decidua (membrane of uterus discarded during menstruation) • deciduate (interlocking of fetal and maternal tissue) • deciduoma (mass of decidual tissue, possibly cancerous)

deciduate—*see* decidua

deciduoma—*see* decidua

decision (judgment; ability to choose) • discission (making an incision)

decrease (reduction) • decrees (legal orders) • degrease (to remove oil or grease) • degrees (units of measure; certificates of higher education; extent)

decrees—*see* decrease

decrement (stage of decline of disease; decrease) • detriment (harm)

deed—*see* dead

defer (to postpone) • differ (to disagree)

deference (respect; submission) • deferens (duct, as in vas deferens) • difference (unlike)

deferens—*see* deference

deficient (defective; lacking in some quality) • deficit (shortfall in quantity, e.g., money)

deficit—*see* deficient

definite (precise; certain) • definitive (conclusive; final)

definitive—*see* definite

defuse (to calm things; to disable an explosive device) • diffuse (to disseminate; to scatter)

degrease—*see* decrease

degrees—*see* decrease

deletion (removal) • delusion (self-deception) • dilatation or dilation (widening)

delude (to deceive) • dilate (to make wider) • dilute (to water down)

delusion—*see* deletion

demote (to reduce one's rank) • denote (to mark or identify)

dengue (date fever, a tropical fever) • dung (animal feces)

denote—*see* demote

dens (a tooth) • dense (thick) • dentes (teeth) • dents (hollows caused by blows or pressure)

dense—*see* dens

dentes—*see* dens

dents—*see* dens

deposition (testimony under oath) • disposition (temperament)

dermatitis (skin inflammation) • dermatosis (skin disease lacking inflammation) • dermostosis (skin tumor)

dermatosis—*see* dermatitis

dermostosis—*see* dermatitis

descendants (people descending from their parents or foreparents) • descendens (a descending structure)

descendens—*see* descendants

descent—*see* decent

desiccant (substance that absorbs moisture) • desiccate (to dry)

desiccate—*see* desiccant

desperate (serious; hopeless) • disparate (different; varied)

detriment—*see* decrement

dexterous or dextrous (skillful) • dextrose (glucose form used in injections)

dextran (plasma volume extender) • dextrin (starch sugar)

dextrin—*see* dextran

dextrose—*see* dexterous or dextrous

dextrous—*see* dexterous

117

diabetic (person with diabetes) •
diabetid or diabetide (skin
disorders caused by diabetes) •
diabrotic (corrosive; ulcer
inducing)

diabetid—*see* diabetic

diabetide—*see* diabetic

diabrotic—*see* diabetic

diaclasis (fracture created to correct
bone deformity) • diaclast
(instrument used on fetus' skull)

diaclast—*see* diaclasis

diacritic (diagnostic; modifying
phonetic marker) • diacritical
(distinguishing; distinctive)

diacritical—*see* diacritic

diad (a pair; a bivalent element) •
died (deceased) • diet (reduced
food intake) • dyed (changed
color)

diagnoses (pl. of *diagnosis*) •
diagnosis (evaluation; analysis)

diagnosis—*see* diagnoses

diagram (plan; sketch) • diaphragm
(membrane; contraceptive device)

diaphragm—*see* diagram

diarrhea (abnormal fecal discharge) •
diarrhemia (excess of blood
plasma)

diarrhemia—*see* diarrhea

diastalsis (contraction in digestive
system) • diastase (enzyme used
to make maltose) • diastasis
(dislocation)

diastase—*see* diastalsis

diastasis—*see* diastalsis

diathetic (pertaining to inborn
disposition toward disease) •
dietetic (relating to diet; food used

in special diets) • dietetics
(scientific study of nutrition)

dicromat (a person with limited color
vision) • dicromate (salt with a
bivalent radical)

dicromate—*see* dicromat

die (to decease; to stop living) • dye
(to stain with different color)

died—*see* diad

diet—*see* diad

dietetic—*see* diathetic

dietetics—*see* diathetic

differ—*see* defer

difference—*see* deference

diffuse—*see* defuse

digitalin (glycocides taken from
digitalis) • digitalis (foxglove leaf
product that includes digitoxin;
cardiac stimulant) • *Digitalis*
(genus of herbs, including
foxglove) • digitoxin (a derivative
of digitalis used in heart failure) •
digoxin (a different digitalis
derivative that increases heart
muscle contraction)

digitalis—*see* digitalin

Digitalis—*see* digitalin

digitoxin—*see* digitalin

digoxin—*see* digitalin

dilate—*see* delude

dilatation—*see* deletion

dilation—*see* deletion

dilute—*see* delude

dilution—*see* delusion

diphtheria (acute infectious disease)
• *Dipteria* (genus of small insects)

Diplodia (genus of fungus that
destroys corn) • diploic (double) •

diploid (with two sets of chromosomes) • **diploidy** (having two sets of chromosomes) • **diplopia** (double vision)

diploic—*see Diplodia*

diploid—*see Diplodia*

diploidy—*see Diplodia*

diplopia—*see Diplodia*

Dipteria—*see* diphtheria

disapprove (to condemn) • **disprove** (to prove false)

disburse (to pay out) • **disperse** (to separate; to send in different directions)

discission—*see* decision

discreet (cautious; able to keep secrets) • **discrete** (discontinuous)

discrete—*see* discreet

discus (disc; round plate) • **discuss** (talk)

discuss—*see* discus

disease—*see* decease

disillusion (to free from false beliefs) • **dissolution** (the break-up of a substance; immersion in liquid)

disinfectant (chemical that destroys harmful microorganisms) • **disinfestant** (chemical that destroys small pests and animals)

disinfestant—*see* disinfectant

disparate—*see* desperate

disperse—*see* disburse

disposition—*see* deposition

disprove—*see* disapprove

dissolution—*see* disillusion

distal (remote) • **distill** (to heat and cool)

distill—*see* distal

diurnal (taking place during the day) • **diurnule** (single pill with a full-day's dose)

diurnule—*see* diurnal

diverticulitis (inflammation of the diverticulum, a sac in the intestinal tract) • **diverticulosis** (existence of a sac in the intestine that is not inflamed)

diverticulosis—*see* diverticulitis

do (to perform; to act) • **due** (owing; scheduled)

does (performs; acts) • **dose** (amount of medication given at one time)

dollar (one hundred cents) • **dolor** (pain; indication of inflammation) • **duller** (more dull; not sharp)

dolor—*see* dollar

donee (recipient of a donation such as blood, money, or an organ) • **donor** (one who gives a donation such as blood, money, or an organ)

donor—*see* donee

dopa (an amino acid, as in L-dopa) • **dope** (slang for illegal drugs)

dope—*see* dopa

dose—*see* does

drops (doses of liquid medicine such as eye drops) • **dropsy** (excess of fluid in tissues)

dropsy—*see* drops

ductal (relating to a channel or tube) • **ductile** (able to be drawn into strands or to be reshaped) • **ductule** (a small duct or tube)

ductile—*see* ductal

ductule—*see* ductal

due—*see* do

duller—*see* dollar

dung—*see* dengue

dye—*see* die

dyed—*see* diad

dyscheria (inability to distinguish which side of body is touched) • dyscholia (a bile disorder) • dyschroia (a bad complexion) • dyschylia (disorder of chyle, an intestinal fluid) • dyscoria (eye pupil abnormality)

dyscholia—*see* dyscheria

dyschroia—*see* dyscheria

dyschylia—*see* dyscheria

dyscoria—*see* dyscheria

dysphagia (difficulty swallowing) • dysphasia (a speech disorder) • dysplasia (abnormal cell or tissue development)

dysphasia—*see* dysphagia

dysplasia—*see* dysphagia

dystonic (relating to diseased muscle tone) • dystopic (misplaced bodily organ)

dystopic—*see* dystonic

E

ecdemic (relates to diseases brought into an area from outside) • endemia (a disease prevalent in an area) • endemic (commonly found in an area) • endermatic or endermic (treatment through the skin) • endyma (membrane lining) • epidemic (rapid spread of infectious disease) • pandemic (epidemic covering several nations)

echocardiogram (record produced by an echocardiograph) • echocardiograph (instrument used to measure motion of heart) • echocardiography (use of ultrasound as heart measuring device) • echography (use of ultrasound as general diagnostic tool)

echocardiograph—*see* echocardiogram

echocardiography—*see* echocardiogram

echography—*see* echocardiogram

echophrasia (patient's repetition of words spoken to him or her) • echopraxia (uncontrolled imitation of other's movements)

echopraxia—*see* echophrasia

ecphoria (revival of memory trace) • euphoria (feeling of well-being; happiness)

ectoderm (outer layers of early embryo) • endoderm or entoderm (inner layers of early embryo)

ectomorph (relatively thin body) • endomorph (relatively fat body)

effect—*see* affect

efferent—*see* afferent

effluent—*see* affluent

egoism (self-interest) • egotism (conceit)

egotism—*see* egoism

either (one of two; also) • **ether** (an anesthetic)

electrocardiogram (the record or tracing produced by an electrocardiograph) • **electrocardiograph** (the instrument used in electrocardiography) • **electrocardiography** (measurement of heart's electric currents)

electrocardiograph—*see* electrocardiogram

electrocardiography—*see* electrocardiogram

electrokymograph (instrument that records changes in organs) • **electromyograph** (instrument used to study skeletal muscle) • **electromyography** (the study of skeletal structures)

electrometrogram (instrument that records uterine contractions) • **electromyogram** (the record of an electromyograph)

electromyogram—*see* electrometrogram

electromyograph—*see* electrokymograph

electromyography—*see* electrokymograph

elementary—*see* alimentary

eluate (material separated by washing) • **elude** (to escape; evade) • **elute** (to separate materials using a solvent)

elude—*see* eluate

elusive (hard to remember; avoiding) • **illusive** (deceptive; of an illusion)

elute—*see* eluate

elution (process of separation by washing) • **illusion** (false belief)

emission (the process of sending out heat, light, gas, etc.) • **omission** (act of leaving out)

enable (to make possible) • **unable** (lacking ability to perform)

encrust or **incrust** (to form a crust) • **incross** (inbred individual)

endemia—*see* ecdemic

endemic—*see* ecdemic

endermatic—*see* ecdemic

endermic—*see* ecdemic

endoderm—*see* ectoderm

endodontics (treatment of teeth roots) • **endodontist** (one who performs endodontics)

endodontist—*see* endodontics

endomorph—*see* ectomorph

endoderm—*see* ectoderm

endyma—*see* ecdemic

enema—*see* anima

enervate (to weaken) • **innervate** (to provide nerves) • **innovate** (to create something new)

entoderm—*see* ectoderm

epidemic—*see* ecdemic

erect (to build, construct) • **eruct** (to belch; to erupt with violence) • **erupt** (to break out suddenly)

erection (swelling of sexual organs in excitation) • **eructation** (belching)

erogenous—*see* aerogenous

erotic (sexually stimulating) • **erotica** (erotic art or literature) • **exotic** (unusual; rare; foreign)

erotica—*see* erotic

eruct—*see* erect

eructation—*see* erection

erupt—*see* erect

erythema—*see* arrhythmia

eschar (a slough; a scab following a burn) • scar (mark left by healing) • scare (to frighten)

estrous or oestrus (pertains to *estrus*) • estrus (animal sexual heat) • *Oestrus* (insects that can cause eye infection)

estrus—*see* estrous

ether—*see* either

ethnology (study of races of humankind) • ethology (study of animals)

ethology—*see* ethnology

eunuch (a castrated male) • unique (only one of its kind)

euphoria—*see* ecphoria

everyday (daily; ordinary) • every day (each separate day)

every day—*see* everyday

everyone (all people in a group or in the world) • every one (each one separately)

every one—*see* everyone

everything (all the things; very important) • every thing (each thing)

every thing—*see* everything

exercise (to engage in regular physical activity; to employ) • exorcise (to drive out evil spirits)

exogenous—*see* axogenous

exon—*see* axon

exorcise—*see* exercise

exotic—*see* erotic

eyed (looked at) • id (unconscious instinctive human drives) • I'd (contr. of *I would*; *I had*)

F

facet (plane on a hard body; side; aspect) • faucet (device to turn water on and off)

facial (pertaining to the face) • fascia (fibrous tissue) • fascial (relating to the fascia) • fascicle (cluster of muscle or nerve fibers)

facies (facial expression) • feces (excrement)

faction (small contentious group in larger organization) • fraction (a chemical constituent that can be separated; a part)

facts (truths; data) • falx (a sickle-shaped structure) • fax (electronic messaging device)

faint (to lose consciousness; very light) • feint (a deceptive move)

fair (light-skinned; impartial) • fare (cost of travel or food)

fallout (nuclear particles; the negative effects of an action) • fall out (to quarrel; to end a relationship)

fall out—*see* fallout

falls (to drop down freely; to lose

one's position) • **false** (not true; misleading)

false—*see* falls

falx—*see* facts

fare—*see* fair

fascia—*see* facial

fascial—*see* facial

fascicle—*see* facial

fatal (deadly; fateful) • **fetal** (relating to the fetus)

fauces (the throat) • **forces** (pressures)

faucet—*see* facet

fax—*see* facts

feat (special achievement) • **feet** (lower extremities)

febrile (feverish) • **feeble** (weak) • **fibril** (a minute fibre)

feces—*see* facies

feeble—*see* febrile

feet—*see* feat

feint—*see* faint

fennel (herb) • **phenyl** (univalent radical)

feral (wild; deadly) • **ferrule** (metal ring applied to tooth)

ferment (to decompose) • **foment** (to instigate)

ferrule—*see* feral

fetal—*see* fatal

fibril—*see* febrile

fibrose (to form fibrous tissues) • **fibrous** (comprising fibers)

fibrous—*see* fibrose

fila (pl. of *filum*; a thin structure) • **filar** (threadlike) • **file** (instrument with serrated edge; to put away

papers in order) • **fill** (to make full; to block, as of a cavity) • **phial** (a small vial)

filar—*see* fila

file—*see* fila

filing (scraping with a file; sorting papers) • **filling** (substance that blocks cavity)

fill—*see* fila

filling—*see* filing

filum (very thin structure) • **phylum** (grouping by ancestry)

fiscal (relating to finances) • **physical** (relating to the body; a medical examination)

fissura (fold in cortex) • **fissure** (deep groove or cleft)

fissure—*see* fissura

fists (hands tightly closed, with fingers bent into palm) • **fits** (seizures; the right size or shape)

fits—*see* fists

flavin (a water-soluble pigment) • **flavine** (a dye used as an antiseptic) • **flavone** (a crystalline used to strengthen capillaries)

flavine—*see* flavin

flavone—*see* flavin

fleas (insects) • **fleece** (interlocking fibers) • **flees** (runs away)

flecks (particles; flakes) • **flex** (to bend)

fleece—*see* fleas

flees—*see* fleas

flew (moved through air; took an airplane) • **flu** (influenza)

flex—*see* flecks

flexor (a muscle that bends a joint) • **flexura** (bent part of a joint or structure) • **flexure** (a bending; a flexura)

flexura—*see* flexor

flexure—*see* flexor

flocks (groups of certain animals) • **flocs** (minute masses of small particles) • **flux** (continuous flow of materials; state of uncertainty and change)

flocs—*see* flocks

floor (base of a room or the base in a measurement) • **fluor** (a discharge)

flu—*see* flew

fluor—*see* floor

fluorane (an intravenous dye) • **fluorene** (a water-soluble substance used to make resins and dyes) • **fluorine** (a toxic gas)

fluorene—*see* fluorane

fluorine—*see* fluorane

flux—*see* flocs

foment—*see* ferment

fool (a stupid person; to deceive) • **fuel** (source of energy, such as gasoline) • **full** (complete; whole)

for (intended to be given; in place of) • **fore** (at the head or top; most important) • **fore-** (prefix meaning *front*) • **four** (the number between three and five)

forces—*see* fauces

fore—*see* for

fore-—*see* fore

forth (forward in time or place) • **fourth** (the position after third)

four—*see* for

fourth—*see* forth

fraction—*see* faction

frays (fights; wears out) • **phrase** (a group of words, less than a sentence, that still conveys meaning)

frees (sets free; releases) • **freeze** (to be or make very cold)

freeze—*see* frees

fucose (an unusual starch found in blood groups) • *Fucus* (a genus of seaweed)

Fucus—*see* fucose

fuel—*see* fool

Fugu (a poisonous Japanese fish) • **fugue** (a loss of conscious awareness of one's acts)

fugue—*see* Fugu

full—*see* fool

furfural or **furfurol** (a fluid obtained from distillation of bran) • **furfuryl** (a radical derived from furfural)

furfurol—*see* furfural

furfuryl—*see* furfural

G

galactan (gelose; produces galactose) • **galactans** (agar carbohydrates)

galactans—*see* galactan

galactase (milk enzyme) • **galactose** (product of lactose hydrolysis)

galactophagous (drinking milk) •

124

galactophygous (halting milk secretion)

galactophygous—*see* galactophagous

galactose—*see* galactase

galea (head bandage) • **galena** (lead sulfide)

galena—*see* galea

gallein (test of fluid reaction) • **gallin** (protamine) • **gallon** (four quarts)

gallin—*see* gallein

gallon—*see* gallein

gastrocele (stomach hernia) • **gastrocoele** (early embryo's cavity)

gastrocoele—*see* gastrocele

Gaultheria (leaf that yields methyl salicylate) • **gaultherin** (a glucoside)

gaultherin—*see Gaultheria*

gauze (light fabric covering) • **gaze** (look; to look at)

gaze—*see* gauze

gelose (galactan) • **gelosis** (mass in tissue)

gelosis—*see* gelose

genial (of the chin) • **genital** (about reproduction)

genital—*see* genial

genius (special intelligence or aptitude) • **genu** (angular structure) • **genus** (classification)

genu—*see* genius

genus—*see* genius

geranial (citral isomer) • **geraniol** (type of alcohol)

geraniol—*see* geranial

geriatrics (treatment of aging) •

geriatrist (geriatrician)

geriatrist—*see* geriatrics

gibbous (humpbacked) • **gibbus** (badly curbed back)

gibbus—*see* gibbous

glands (fluid-secreting organs) • **glans** (small round masses)

glandula (special secreting cells) • **glandular** (pertaining to a gland or to the glans penis)

glandular—*see* glandula

glans—*see* glands

globi (granular bodies) • **globin** (histone)

globin—*see* globi

glucase (enzyme helping to make glucose) • **glucose** (grape sugar)

glucose—*see* glucase

gluten (grain protein) • **glutin** (gelatin; viscid substance)

glutin—*see* gluten

glycine (an amino acid) • **Glycine** (type of legume)

Glycine—*see* glycine

glycogenesis (making of glycogen) • **glycogenosis** (error in making glycogen)

glycogenosis—*see* glycogenesis

gnosia (ability to know nature) • **nausea** (vomity feeling)

gonial (relating to a point on the mandible) • **gonidial** (parts of a lichen)

gonidial—*see* gonial

gonion (point of lower jawbone) • **gonium** (relating to sexual organs)

gonium—*see* gonion

graft (new part to remedy defect) •
graphed (made data presentation)

gram (unit of mass) • **Gram**
(bacteriologist; Gram's stain)

Gram—*see* gram

granula (small particle; related to
nigroid body) • **granular** (made
up of particles) • **granule** (small
grain or particle)

granular—*see* granula

granule—*see* granula

graphed—*see* graft

gravid (pregnant) • **gravida** (pregnant
woman)

gravida—*see* gravid

gravidity (state of pregnancy) •
gravity (weight, density)

gravity—*see* gravidity

grip (grasp) • **gripe** (colic; complaint)
• **grippe** (flu)

gripe—*see* grip

grippe—*see* grip

gut (intestine, catgut) • **gutta** (liquid
drop) • **gutter** (bone incision) •
guttur (throat)

gutta—*see* gut

gutter—*see* gut

guttur—*see* gut

gyrosa (like vertigo) • **gyrose**
(denoting irregular curved lines) •
gyrus (brain elevation)

gyrose—*see* gyrosa

gyrus—*see* gyrosa

H

habit (a regular, automatic way of
acting) • **habitat** (natural
environment)

habitat—*see* habit

habitual (customary; usual) •
habituate (to become accustomed
to)

habituate—*see* habitual

hairy (full of hair) • **harry** (to
pressure; bother)

half (one of two equal parts) • **halve**
(to cut in half; to divide equally) •
halves (pl. of *half*) • **have** (to
possess)

halve—*see* half

halves—*see* half

hamartoma (a benign nodule) •
hematoma (a blood clot)

hamulus (a hook-like structure or
process) • **humerus** (bone of the
upper arm) • **humulus** (hops used
as a poultice)

hang-up (inhibition or problem) •
hang up (to end a phone
conversation)

hang up—*see* hang-up

Hansen (physician; Hansen bacillus)
• **Hanson** (surgeon; Hanson's unit)
• **Hensen** (anatomist; Hensen's
canal)

Hanson—*see* Hansen

hard (tough; difficult) • **heart**

(central bodily organ that pumps blood)

harry—*see* hairy

haunch (part of the buttocks) • **hunch** (intuition, feeling)

have—*see* half

head (top of the body; the mind; top person in organization) • **he'd** (contr. of *he had* or *he would*) • **heed** (to pay attention; to agree)

heal (to make one healthy) • **heel** (back of the foot) • **he'll** (contr. of *he will*)

hear (to detect sound) • **here** (at this place)

heart—*see* hard

he'd—*see* head

heed—*see* head

heel—*see* heal

heinous—*see* anise

helico- (prefix for a *relationship to a coil*) • **helio-** (prefix denoting a *relationship to the sun*)

helio-—*see* helico

he'll—*see* heal

hematein (crystalline substance used as a stain) • **hematin** (an iron constituent of hemoglobin)

hematin—*see* hematein

hematoma—*see* hamartoma

hematophagous (blood drinking) • **hematophagus** (blood-sucking insect)

hematophagus—*see* hematophagous

hemihyperesthesia (abnormal increase in feeling on one side of the body) • **hemihypesthesia** (abnormal decrease in feeling on one side of the body)

hemihypesthesia—*see* hemihyperesthesia

hemogeneous (of blood circulation) • **homogeneous** (similar)

hemometer (instrument that measures hemoglobin) • **hemometra** (blood accumulation in the uterus)

hemometra—*see* hemometer

hemophilia (hereditary blood disease) • **hemophiliac** (person with hemophilia) • **hemophilic** (possessing an affinity for blood)

hemophiliac—*see* hemophilia

hemophilic—*see* hemophilia

hemophobia (deep fear of blood or bleeding) • **homophobia** (irrational fear of homosexuals)

Hensen—*see* Hansen

here—*see* hear

heterologous (comprised of abnormal tissue) • **heteronomous** (of different laws of growth) • **heteronymous** (opposite) • **homologous** (analogous)

heteronomous—*see* heterologous

heteronymous—*see* heterologous

heterotopia (misplacement of body parts) • **heterotrophia** (a nutritional disorder) • **heterotropia** (a visual defect)

heterotrophia—*see* heterotopia

heterotropia—*see* heterotopia

high-grade (high quality) • **high grade** (a good mark or score)

high grade—*see* high-grade

histoma (a fibroma; tumor) • **histone** (a simple protein that often indicates a blood disease) • **histotone** (a cutting instrument)

histone—*see* histoma

histotone—*see* histoma

Hodgkin's disease (malignancy with multiple characteristics) • Hodgson's disease (a heart disease)

Hodgson's disease—*see* Hodgkin's disease

hole (an opening; a gap) • whole (complete; entire)

homocysteine (product of methionine) • homocystine (source of sulphur)

homocystine—*see* homocysteine

homogeneous—*see* hemogeneous

homologous—*see* heterologous

homophobia—*see* hemophobia

hour (60 minutes) • our (belongs to us)

human (a person) • humane (with compassion)

humane—*see* human

humeral (of the upper arm bone) • humoral (of bodily fluids)

humerus—*see* hamulus

humoral—*see* humeral

humulene (a hydrocarbon) • humulin (sedative granular powder)

humulin—*see* humulene

humulus—*see* hamulus

hunch—*see* haunch

hydrastine (an alkaloid) • hydrastinine (an artificial alkaloid)

hydrastinine—*see* hydrastine

hypercholesterolemia (excess blood cholesterol) • hypercholesterolia (excess bile secretion)

hypercholesterolia—*see* hypercholesterolemia

hyperglycemia (excess blood sugar) • hyperglycinemia (excess blood glycine) • hypoglycemia (shortage of blood sugar)

hyperglycinemia—*see* hyperglycemia

hypertension (high blood pressure) • hypotension (low blood pressure)

hyperthermia (high body temperature) • hypothermia (low temperature)

hypoglycemia—*see* hyperglycemia

hypotension—*see* hypertension

hypothermia—*see* hyperthermia

hysterotrachelectomy (amputation of the uteri of the cervix) • hysterotrachelotomy (incision of the uteri of the cervix)

hysterotrachelotomy—*see* hysterotrachelectomy

I

id—*see* eyed

I'd—*see* eyed

ileac (of the ileum) • iliac (relating to hipbone)

iliac—*see* ileac

illusion—*see* elution

illusive—*see* elusive

imbalance (lack of balance) • in balance (in equilibrium)

in balance—*see* imbalance

incisor (an anterior tooth) • **incisura** or **incisure** (notch or cut)

incisura—*see* incisor

incisure—*see* incisor

incross—*see* encrust or incrust

incrust—*see* encrust

infarction (death of organ or part) • **infraction** (bone fracture)

infer- (to conclude; prefix indicating *below* or *lower*) • **infra-** (prefix indicating *beneath*)

infra-—*see* infer-

infraction—*see* infarction

innervate—*see* enervate

innovate—*see* enervate

interface (common surface or boundary) • **interphase** (cell division interval)

intermission (interval) • **intromission** (insertion of one part into another)

intern (to gain professional experience in hospital; to confine) • **interne** or **intern** (hospital resident) • **in turn** (in order)

interne—*see* intern

interphase—*see* interface

intervenous (between veins) • **intravenous** (within or into a vein)

intravenous—*see* intervenous

intromission—*see* intermission

in turn—*see* intern

irremeable (cannot return) • **irremediable** (incurable)

irremediable—*see* irremeable

J-K

Jansen (otologist) • **Jensen** (chemist and classifier)

Jensen—*see* Jansen

keratosis (skin's horny growth) • **ketosis** (high levels of ketone)

ketosis—*see* keratosis

L

labial (of the lips of tooth surface; of the labia) • **labile** (gliding; chemically unstable)

labile—*see* labial

lacrimal (pertaining to tears) • **lacrimale** (point in skull)

lacrimale—*see* lacrimal

lacuna (small depression) • **lacunar** (pertaining to lacuna or a hiatus of a symptom)

lacunar—*see* lacuna

lamina (thin tissue layer) • **laminar** (arranged in plates or layers)

laminar—*see* lamina

lanced (cut) • **lancet** (surgical knife)

lancet—*see* lanced

Lange (excess globulin method) • **Langer** (anatomist; muscles, arches) • **languor** (weakness; listlessness)

Langer—*see* Lange

Langerhans' (cells, islands) • **Langhans** (pathologist; cell research)

Langhans—*see* Langerhans'

languor—*see* Lange

laser (strong light beams) • **lazar** (leper)

lazar—*see* laser

leach (to separate soluble parts) • **leche** (sap or milk) • **leech** (sucking worm)

leche—*see* leach

leech—*see* leach

leper (one having leprosy, Hansen's disease) • **lepra** (aggravation of skin lumps)

lepra—*see* leper

leucine (amino acid) • **leukin** (lytic substance)

leukin—*see* leucine

lie (untruth) • **lye** (alkaline used in soap)

ligament (bone-linking tissue) • **ligamenta** (bands joining carpal bones)

ligamenta—*see* ligament

linea (ridge or streak) • **lineae** (pl. of *linea*) • **linear** (like a line)

lineae—*see* linea

linear—*see* linea

linen (flax cloth) • **linin** (material in cell nucleus)

lingual (of the tongue) • **lingula** (tongue-like structure)

lingula—*see* lingual

linin—*see* linen

linoleic (fatty acid) • **linolenic** (pertaining to a colorless liquid) • **linolic** (pertaining to fatty acids)

linolenic—*see* linoleic

linolic—*see* linoleic

lipa (relating to fatty acids) • **lippa** (ciliaris)

lippa—*see* lipa

lips (fleshy folds of mouth) • **lisps** (mispronounces s, z)

lisps—*see* lips

liter (metric measure of volume) • **litter** (stretcher; to give birth; to scatter trash)

litter—*see* liter

liver (large critical gland in abdominal cavity) • **livor** (post-death discoloration)

livor—*see* liver

lobes (rounded part of organ) • **lobus** (subdivisions of organs)

lobule (clear subdivisions of organs) • **lobuli** (pl. of *lobule*)

lobuli—*see* lobule

lobus—*see* lobes

local (one area or location) • **lochial** (pertaining to vaginal discharges)

lochial—*see* local

loop (bend in tubular organs) • **loupe** (special viewing lens)

loose (not tight) • **lues** (infectious disease, specifically syphilis)

loupe—*see* loop

lues—*see* loose

luminal (pertaining to a tubular cavity) • **Luminal** (phenobarbital)

Luminal—*see* luminal

lycine (betaine) • **lysin** (antibody) • **lysine** (amino acid)

lye—*see* lie

lyosol (liquid dispersal medium) • **Lysol** (disinfectant)

lysin—*see* lycine

lysine—*see* lycine

Lysol—*see* lyosol

M

macrocephalous (unusually large head) • **macrocephalus** (a person with unusually large head)

macrocephalus—*see* macrocephalous

macrodactilia (abnormally large toes and fingers) • **macrodactyly** (state of having abnormally sized digits)

macrodactyly—*see* macrodactilia

macula (a stain or discoloration) • **macular** (having stain or discoloration) • **macule** (patch of skin altered in color, a sign of various diseases)

macular—*see* macula

macule—*see* macula

mal (disease; sickness) • **Mall** (anatomist; formula re: age of human embryo)

maladie (a disease attached to a specific illness) • **malady** (any disease)

malady—*see* maladie

malaria (mosquito-caused illness) • **miliaria** (prickly heat) • **miliary** (having lesions like millet seeds)

Mall—*see* mal

maltase (an enzyme) • **maltose** (a sugar)

maltose—*see* maltase

man (adult male; human) • **Mann** (U. S. surgeon; U test)

mandrel or **mandril** (dental tool shaft) • **mandrill** (a baboon)

mandril—*see* mandrel

mandrill—*see* mandrel

Mann—*see* man

massage (body rub) • **message** (communication)

mastoplasia (breast tissue development) • **mastoplastia** (abnormal breast tissue)

mastoplastia—*see* mastoplasia

mastostomy (breast incision for drainage) • **mastotomy** (any incision of the breast)

mastotomy—*see* mastostomy

materia (matter) • **material** (base for concept; object)

material—*see* materia

measle (tapeworm, larva) • **measles** (respiratory viral infection) • **measly** (containing tapeworms)

measles—*see* measle

measly—*see* measle

Medicaid (medical care for the poor)

• **medicate** (to provide medication)

medicate—*see* Medicaid

megalomaniac (person with delusions of grandeur) • **megalomanic** (having delusions of grandeur)

megalomanic—*see* megalomaniac

megalopia (abnormally large eyes) • **megalopsia** (vision disturbance)

megalopsia—*see* megalopia

meiosis (cell division) • **miosis** (eye pupil constriction)

melancholia (depression) • **melancholiac** (a depressed person) • **melancholic** (depressed; relating to melancholia)

melancholiac—*see* melancholia

melancholic—*see* melancholia

membrana (a thin skin; membrane) • **membrane** (thin tissue lining or surrounding body parts)

membrane—*see* membrana

menstruation (periodic discharge from the uterus) • **mensuration** (the process or act of measuring)

mensuration—*see* menstruation

menthol (a mint-based alcohol) • **menthyl** (a radical with a valent of one)

menthyl—*see* menthol

mesoglea (layer beneath epidermis) • **mesoglia** (neurological cell)

mesoglia—*see* mesoglea

mesothelia (embryo cell layers) • **mesothelial** (concerning the mesothelia)

mesothelial—*see* mesothelia

mesovarian (holding the ligament of the ovary) • **mesovarium** (the ligament that holds the ovary)

mesovarium—*see* mesovarian

message—*see* massage

metamer (similar isomers) • **metamere** (animal body part)

metamere—*see* metamer

metamorphose (to change form; to degenerate) • **metamorphosis** (a change of form)

metamorphosis—*see* metamorphose

metastases—*see* metastasis

metastasis (movement of cancer cells from original site to another part of the body) • **metastases** (pl. of *metastasis*)

Metazoa (division of the animal kingdom, excluding Protozoa) • **metazoal** (relating to the multi-cellular animal kingdom)

Metazoal—*see* metazoa

methanal (formaldehyde) • **methanol** (a flammable liquid)

methanol—*see* methanal

methene (bivalent radical) • **methine** (a radical of wood alcohol)

methine—*see* methene

metopion (point in forehead) • **metopium** (anterior of brain's frontal lobe) • **metopon** (a morphine derivative)

metopium—*see* metopion

metopon—*see* metopion

microcephalous (with a small head) • **microcephalus** (a person with small head)

microcephalus—*see* microcephalous

microglia (neurological cells) •

microglial (pertaining to microglia)

microglial—*see* microglia

miliaria—*see* malaria

miliary—*see* malaria

minimum (least, smallest) • **minium** (reddish lead oxide)

minium—*see* minimum

minor (unimportant) • **Minor** (Russian neurologist)

Minor—*see* minor

miosis—*see* meiosis

misogamy (aversion to marriage) • misogyny (hatred of women)

misogyny—*see* misogamy

mobility (facility of movement) • motility (ability to move spontaneously)

modal (of a statistical measure) • model (dentist cast; example)

model—*see* modal

mold (fungous growth; wax-pressed cast) • **molt** (to shed; to cast off)

molt—*see* mold

Monilia (fruit molds) • **monilial** (pertains to *Monilia*, but often refers to *Candida*)

monilial—*see* Monilia

monochromat (a person who is color blind) • **monochromate** (relating to one color)

monochromate—*see* monochromat

monogamy (marriage to one person at a time) • **monogony** (nonsexual reproduction)

monogeny (a sexual reproduction; descent from a common pair) • monogyny (marriage with one wife; having one style)

monogony—*see* monogamy

monogyny—*see* monogeny

monophagia (wanting only one food or one meal a day) • **monophasia** (speaking only one word or phrase)

monophasia—*see* monophagia

morphea (cutaneous lesions) • morphia (morphine)

morphia—*see* morphea

motility—*see* mobility

mucous (pertaining to a mucus discharge) • **mucus** (discharge issuing from mucus membranes)

mucus—*see* mucous

myatonia (lacking muscle tone) • myotonia (muscle rigidity)

myotactic (of muscular sense) • myotatic (re: muscle stretching)

myotatic—*see* myotactic

myotonia—*see* myatonia

N

naevose or nevose (marked by nevi) • nevus (a birthmark)

nausea—*see* gnosia

necrotic (relating to death of a tissue) • neurotic (suffering from or pertaining to a neurosis) •

neurotica (functional nervous disorders)

Nematoda (parasites like roundworms) • nematode (any parasitic worm)

nematode—see Nematoda

nerve (tissue connecting parts of nervous system) • nervi (pl. of nervus; fascicles)

nervi—see nerve

nervous (apprehensive; jumpy) • nervus (nerve fibers)

nervus—see nervous

neurilemma (wrapping for myelin layers) • neurilemmal (the quality of enwrapping myelin)

neurilemmal—see neurilemma

neurosyphilid (having syphilis of nervous system) • neurosyphilis (syphilis of central nervous system)

neurosyphilis—see neurosyphilid

neurotic—see necrotic

neurotica—see necrotic

nevose—see naevose

nevus—see naevose

nitrate (a salt or nitric acid) • nitride (a compound of nitrogen and a metal) • nitrite (nitrous acid salt)

nitride—see nitrate

nitrite—see nitrate

node (swelling or knot) • nodi (pl. of node or nodus)

nodi—see node

nodose (swollen) • nodus (a node)

nodus—see nodose

noma (gangrene of mouth) • nona (encephalitis-like disease)

nona—see noma

O

octan (every eighth day) • octane (oily hydrocarbon)

octane—see octan

od (force of magnets on nervous system) • odd (peculiar)

odd—see od

oestrus—see estrous

Oestrus—see estrous

oligogenic (referring to certain hereditary characteristics produced by a few genes at most) • oligogenics (birth control)

oligogenics—see oligogenic

omission—see emission

oncology (study of tumors) • ontology (a branch of philosophy)

ontology—see oncology

ora (the mouth; an uneven edge) • oral (by or of the mouth) • orale (point in alveolar process)

oral—see aural; ora

orale—see ora

orbital (pertaining to the eyeball cavity) • orbitale (orbit's inferior margin)

orbitale—see orbital

orchidotomy or **orchiotomy** or
orchotomy (incision into the
testes) • **orchiectomy** (excision of
a testis)

orchiectomy—*see* orchidotomy

orchiotomy—*see* orchidotomy

orchotomy—*see* orchidotomy

orthoptic (correcting slantic vision) •
orthotic (serving to protect or
improve a function) • **orthotopic**
(occurring in a normal place) •
orthotropic (growing vertically)

orthotic—*see* orthoptic

orthotopic—*see* orthoptic

orthotropic—*see* orthoptic

osteologia (nomenclature of bones) •
osteology (study of bones)

osteology—*see* osteologia

ostia (orifices, openings) • **ostial**
(pertaining to an opening)

ostial—*see* ostia

our—*see* hour

ova (female reproductive cells; pl. of
ovum) • **oval** (egg-shaped) • **over**
(above)

oval—*see* ova

over—*see* ova

ovoid—*see* avoid

P

palpate (to examine by touch) •
palpitate (to beat rapidly)

palpation (act of examining with
hands) • **palpitation** (increased
heart beat)

palpitate—*see* palpate

palpitation—*see* palpation

pandemic—*see* ecdemic

pannus (corneal tissue covering) •
panus (lymphatic gland
inflammation)

pantaphobia (lacking fear) •
pantophobia (fearing everything)

pantophobia—*see* pantaphobia

panus—*see* pannus

papilla (a small, nipple-like
projection) • **papula** (small skin
elevation) • **papular** (with a
papule) • **papule** (a small papula)

pappose (having downy surface) •
pappus (first beard growth)

pappus—*see* pappose

papula—*see* papilla

papular—*see* papilla

papule—*see* papilla

paracyesis (ectopic pregnancy) •
paresis (partial paralysis)

paracytic (among cells) • **parasitic**
(living at expense of another
organism)

paraglossa (swelling of the tongue) •
paraglossia (inflammation under
the tongue)

paraglossia—*see* paraglossa

parameter (a limit or boundary) •
perimeter (instrument for eye
examination; outer edge of area)

parasite (one that lives off of others) • pericyte (elongated cell)

parasitic—*see* paracytic

paresis—*see* paracyesis

partes (pl. of *pars*; a division) • parts (subdivision of a portion)

parts—*see* partes

passed (evacuated; voided) • past (ended; gone by) • paste (semisolid mix)

past—*see* passed

paste—*see* passed

patella (sesamoid bone) • patellar (relating to the patella)

patellar—*see* patella

patent (open; obvious) • patient (awaiting medical care; forebearing)

patient—*see* patent

patten (metallic foot support) • pattern (characteristic traits; design)

pattern—*see* patten

paunch (a protruding belly) • punch (an instrument for perforating)

peak (upper limit; highest point) • peek (to look quickly; to glance) • pique (to arouse; to provoke; anger)

pecten (comblike structure) • pectin (fruit substance)

pectin—*see* pecten

pectous (resembling pectin) • pectus (breast or chest)

pectus—*see* pectous

pediculous (infested with lice) • pediculus (a louse; stemlike structure)

pediculus—*see* pediculous

peek—*see* peak

pellicula (epidermis) • pellicular (having a thin skin)

pellicular—*see* pellicula

pelves (pl. of *pelvis*) • pelvis (basinlike structure in lower trunk) • pulvis (powder)

pelvis—*see* pelves

per (a rate; for) • pure (uncontaminated) • purr (vibratory sound)

perfusion (pouring through) • profusion (state of abundance)

pericyte—*see* parasite

perimeter—*see* parameter

perinatal (relating to time of birth) • prenatal (before birth)

perineal (relating to the pelvic floor) • peritoneal (relating to the peritoneum) • peroneal (relating to the side of the leg)

peritoneal—*see* perineal

peroneal—*see* perineal

personal (private; individual) • personnel (employees)

personnel—*see* personal

pervious (permeable) • previous (before)

pes (foot) • pest (plague; insect)

pest—*see* pes

petrosa (hard part of temporal bone) • petrosal (pertaining to petrosa)

petrosal—*see* petrosa

phalangeal (relating to the phalanx) • pharyngeal (relating to the pharynx) pharyngeal—*see* phalangeal

phenyl—*see* fennel

phial—*see* fila

phlegm (mucus) • phloem (plant vascular bundle)

phloem—*see* phlegm

phonation (production of sounds) • pronation (rotation of anatomical parts of the body)

phosphene (sensation of light) • phosphine (gas)

phosphine—*see* phosphene

photogen (phosphorescent microorganism) • photogene (retinal after-image)

photogene—*see* photogen

phrase—*see* frays

phylum—*see* filum

physiatrics (physiotherapy) • physiatrist (specialist in physical medicine)

physiatrist—*see* physiatrics

physic (a cathartic; to purge) • physique (structure and appearance of the body) • psychic (mental)

physical—*see* fiscal

physique—*see* physic

pia (tender) • pial (relating to pia mater)

pial—*see* pia

pilose (hairy) • pilus (hair; light epidermal tissue)

pilus—*see* pilose

pique—*see* peak

planta (sole of foot) • plantar (relating to the sole)

plantar—*see* planta

-plasm (suffix indicating *formative substance*) • plasma (blood's fluid portion)

plasma—*see* -plasm

pleural (relating to the thorax) • plural (pertaining to more than one)

pleuritic (relating to pleurisy) • pruritic (marked by itching)

plural—*see* pleural

pocked (marked with smallpox lesions) • pocket (saclike cavity)

pocket—*see* pocked

pocks (pustules) • pox (viral pustular disease)

poison (damaging, ingested substance) • Poisson (statistician who created probability function)

Poisson—*see* poison

poles (points at extremities of axis) • polus (a pole; one of two extreme points)

polus—*see* poles

polypous (relating to presence of polyps) • polypus (polyp)

polypus—*see* polypous

pore (sweat gland opening) • pour (to cause liquid to flow)

porous (having openings that pass through substances) • porus (a pore or foramen)

porus—*see* porous

pour—*see* pore

pox—*see* pocks

prenatal—*see* perinatal

pressor (raising blood pressure) • pressure (force; measure of force) pressure—*see* pressor

previous—*see* pervious

principal (main) • principle (belief; value)

principle—*see* principal

profusion—*see* perfusion

pronation—*see* phonation

propane (colorless gas) • propene (propylene)

propene—*see* propane

prostate (urethral gland) • prostrate (lacking vitality; prone)

prostrate—*see* prostate

protean (able to change form) • protein (complex nitrogenous compound)

protein—*see* protean

proteose (protein derivative) • proteus (microorganism)

proteus—*see* proteose

Protozoa (simplest organisms of the animal kingdom) • protozoal (about protozoa)

protozoal—*see Protozoa*

pruritic—*see* pleuritic

Prussak (Russian otologist) • prussic (hydrocyanic [in acid])

prussic—*see* Prussak

psychic—*see* physic

psychosis (mental disorder) • sycosis

(inflammation of hair follicles)

psyllium—*see* cilium

pterin (nitrogenous compound) • pterion (sphenoid bone junction)

pterion—*see* pterin

pubes (pl. of *pubis*) • pubis (one of the bones of the pelvic girdle)

pubis—*see* pubes

pulp (soft and juicy tissue) • pulpa (dental pulp) • pulpal (relating to pulp) • pupil (center of iris)

pulpa—*see* pulp

pulpal—*see* pulp

pulvis—*see* pelves

punch—*see* paunch

pupil—*see* pulp

pure—*see* per

purr—*see* per

pyogenes (pus formations) • pyogens (pus-forming agents)

pyogenic (producing pus) • pyrogenic (relating to fever)

pyogens—*see* pyogenes

pyrectic (fever-causing agent) • pyretic (about the nature of fever)

pyretic—*see* pyrectic

pyrexia (fever) • pyrexial (pertaining to fever)

pyrexial—*see* pyrexia

pyrogenic—*see* pyogenic

Q

Quincke (German physician; edema, puncture) • quinque (five)

quinque—*see* Quincke

R

rabbit—*see* rabid

rabid (having rabies) • rabbit (a small mammal)

radian (eye examination measure) • radiant (emanating rays)

radiant—*see* radian

radical (aimed at root cause; group of atoms) • radicle (small branch of nerve or vessel)

radicle—*see* radical

radiobe (radium condensation) • radiode (radium container)

radiode—*see* radiobe

raffinase (enzyme) • raffinose (melitose)

raffinose—*see* raffinase

raise (to elevate) • rays (radiation lines) • raze (to destroy) • Reye's (a syndrome)

ramose (with many branches) • ramus (a branch)

ramus—*see* ramose

rasion (the grating of drugs) • ration (fixed quota; allowance)

raspatory (surgical file) • respiratory (relating to breathing)

ration—*see* rasion

rays—*see* raise

raze—*see* raise

re (regarding) • re- (prefix to indicate *again*) • Re (rhenium) • Rh (rhodium; rhesus factor) • rhe (measure of fluidity)

re-—*see* re

Re—*see* re

reagent (addition to complex solution) • reagin (an antibody)

reagin—*see* reagent

recess (cavity) • recessus (potential spaces)

recessus—*see* recess

record (registration, in dental practice; to write down) • Ricord (French physician; syphilis treatment)

rectostomy (artificial rectal opening) • rectotomy (rectal incision)

rectotomy—*see* rectostomy

reefer (slang for a *marijuana cigarette*) • refer (to direct; to submit for decision)

refer—*see* reefer

reflects (thinks; mirrors) • reflex (automatic response) • reflux (regurgitation)

reflex—*see* reflects

reflux—*see* reflects

regio (limited area of body) • region (area; organ part with special function)

region—*see* regio

relevant (pertinent) • revellent (revulsive)

relief (easing of distress) • relieve (to mitigate; to have a bladder or bowel movement)

relieve—*see* relief

renin (enzyme released by kidney) • rennin (enzyme that coagulates milk)

rennin—*see* renin

repositor (instrument used in displacement) • repository (storage place; location of long-term drug injection)

repository—*see* repositor

residual (left behind; remainder) • residue (nontoxic protein product)

residue—*see* residual

respiratory—*see* raspatory

reticulose (having crossing veins) • reticulosis (malignant growth of lymphatic glands)

reticulosis—*see* reticulose

retina (part of the eyeball) • Retin-A (tretinoin, used to reduce wrinkles) • retinal (related to the retina; a vitamin A derivative that acts on the retina)

Retin-A—*see* retina

retinal—*see* retina

retrocolic (behind the colon) • retrocollic (of the back of the neck)

retrocollic—*see* retrocolic

revellent—*see* relevant

Reye's— *see* raise

Rh—*see* Re

rhamnose (urine excretion) • Rhamnus (shrub)

Rhamnus—*see* rhamnose

rhe—*see* Re

rheum (watery discharge from nose or eyes) • Rheum (a genus of herbs) • room (a space within a building)

Rheum—*see* rheum

rickets (rachitis; infant's disease) • Rickettsia (rod-shaped organisms)

Rickettsia—*see* rickets

Ricord—*see* record

ridged (having a projection) • rigid (stiff; fixed)

right (on the side away from the heart) • rite (a ritual) • write (to inscribe words on paper or a computer)

rigid—*see* ridged

rite—*see* right

Rollet (French syphilis specialist) • Rollett (irrigation device)

Rollett—*see* Rollet

room—*see* rheum

root (portion of organ in tissue) • route (method of transmitting a disease or introducing medicine into the body)

rosein (antibiotics) • rosin (resin used in plasters)

roselle (tropical plant) • roseola (red rash)

roseola—*see* roselle

rosin—*see* rosein

route—*see* root

Roux (bacteriologist; serum) • rue (poisonous herb)

rubber (elastic, solid substance) • ruber (red nucleus) • rubor (redness of the skin)

rubella (German measles) • rubeola (measles)

rubeola—*see* rubella

ruber—*see* rubber

rubor—*see* rubber

rue—*see* Roux

S

sac (a soft-walled anatomical cavity)
• sack (a woven bag)

saccharin (low-calorie sweetener) •
saccharine (relating to sugar)

saccharine—see saccharin

saccule or sacculus (small sac) •
sacculi (smaller sacs of vestibular
labyrinth; pl. of sacculus)

sacculi—see saccule

sacculus—see saccule

Sachs (neurologist; degeneration) •
sacs (pouches)

sack—see sac

sacs—see Sachs

salve (substance for application to
sores or wounds) • Salvia (genus
of plant yielding astringent oil) •
save (to rescue from danger; to
keep intact)

Salvia—see salve

sanatory (salubrious) • sanitary
(promoting health; of sewage
disposal)

sanitary—see sanatory

save—see salve

saw (a device used to cut bone) •
soor (thrush) • sore (a wound; an
ulcer; a lesion; painful)

scapula (shoulder blade) • scapular
(about the shoulder blade)

scapular—see scapula

scar—see eschar

scare—see eschar

scatoma (fecal mass) • scotoma
(depressed vision)

scirrhous—see cirrus

scirrhous—see cirrus

sclerose (to harden) • sclerous
(indurated; hard)

sclerous—see sclerose

scotoma—see scatoma

secreta (products of secretion) •
secrete (to deliver to cell)

secrete—see secreta

secretin (polypeptide hormone) •
secretion (glandular creation)

secretion—see secretin

sella (saddle-like depression) • sellar
(relating to sphenoid bone
depression)

sellar—see sella

semen (sperm) • Semon
(laryngologist)

Semon—see semen

senses—see census

sensor—see censor

serial—see cereal

serious—see cereous

serous—see cirrus

serrated—see cerated

serum—see cerumen

sheath (a covering structure) •
sheathe (to provide covering)

sheathe—see sheath

shoddy (poor quality) • shotty
(granular)

shotty—see shoddy

sight—see cite

sign (indication of abnormality) • **sine** (trigonometric function)

silicon (nonmetallic element) • **silicone** (plastic)

silicone—*see* silicon

simulate (to imitate; malinger) • **stimulate** (to arouse)

sine—*see* sign

sinuous (winding) • **sinus** (hollow; blood passage)

sinus—*see* sinuous

site—*see* cite

sitology—*see* cytology

sol (colloid dispersion; abbrev. for *solution*) • **sole** (bottom of foot; only) • **soul** (spiritual part of a person)

sole—*see* sol

soma (body of an organism) • **stoma** (a small opening) • **stroma** (supporting tissues of an organ) • **struma** (goiter)

soor—*see* saw

sore—*see* saw

soul—*see* sol

spatia (limited areas) • **spatial** (about space)

spatial—*see* spatia

sphygmomanometer (a machine that measures blood pressure) • **sphygmometer** (a machine that measures pulse)

sphygmometer—*see* sphygmomanometer

spicula (pl. of *spicule*) • **spicule** (needle-shaped body)

spicule—*see* spicula

squama (body structure resembling a plate or scale) • **squame** (a flake of skin)

squame—*see* squama

stabile (stable serum; a stationary electrode) • **stable** (steady)

stable—*see* stabile

staff (employees) • **staph** (shortened form of staphylococcus)

staph—*see* staff

stat (immediately) • **-stat** (combining form meaning causing inhibition of growth) • **state** (condition)

-stat—*see* stat

state—*see* stat

stearoyl (the radical of stearic acid) • **sterile** (inability to conceive) • **sterol** (solid alcohol)

stella (star, star-shaped) • **stellar** (outstanding; relating to stars)

stellar—*see* stella

sterile—*see* stearoyl

sterol—*see* stearoyl

stimulate—*see* simulate

stoma—*see* soma

stoop (to crouch; to bend the body forward) • **stupe** (a medicated cloth or sponge) • **stupp** (a poisonous soot)

stricture (narrowing of a body part) • **structure** (an anatomical part arranged in a pattern)

strip (to press or excise) • **stripe** (streak or band)

stripe—*see* strip

stroma—*see* soma

structure—*see* stricture

struma—*see* soma

stupe—*see* stoop

stupp—*see* stoop

sublime (to sublimate; to vaporize and condense) • subline (above and slightly below)

subline—*see* sublime

substantia (substance) • substantial (ample)

substantial—*see* substantia

succus (secretion) • succuss (to shake up)

succuss—*see* succus

sucrase (enzyme used in hydrolysis of sucrose) • sucrose (cane sugar)

sucrose—*see* sucrase

sulfa (any sulfanomide drug) • sulfo- (chemical prefix for divalent sulfur compounds) • sulfur (skin ointment; antioxident; laxative)

sulfo-—*see* sulfa

sulfur—*see* sulfa

sycosis—*see* psychosis

synapse (nerve impulse transmission point) • synapsis (chromosome pairing)

synapsis—*see* synapse

T

tache (freckle, spot) • taches (blemishes)

taches—*see* tache

tachyphagia (rapid eating) • tachyphasia (rapid speech)

tachyphasia—*see* tachyphagia

taenia (a tapeworm) • *Taenia* (special tapeworm genus)

Taenia—*see* taenia

talose (glucose isomer) • talus (ankle bone)

talus—*see* talose

tamarin (primate) • tamarind (laxative fruit pulp)

tamarind—*see* tamarin

tampan (a tick) • tampon (secretion absorber)

tampon—*see* tampan

taper (to diminish gradually) • tapir (mammal whose fat is used as medicine)

tapir—*see* taper

tare (chemical control vessel) • tear (pron. *tayre*: to rip)

tear (pron. *teer*: fluid from eye) • tere (to rub)

tear—*see* tare

tears (fluids from eye) • teres (round, long muscles) • tiers (layers)

technic (technology) • technique (special method; skill)

technique—*see* technic

teeth (pl. of *tooth*) • teethe (to cut one's first teeth)

teethe—*see* teeth

tela (layer of tissue) • teller (a narrator; a person who counts)

teller—*see* tela

tempora (pertaining to the temples) • **temporal** (time limited, temporary)

temporal—*see* tempora

tenderness (sensitivity to touch or palpation) • **tendinous** or **tentinous** (relating to or consisting of a tendon)

tendinitis or **tendonitis** (inflammation of tendon) • **tenonitis** (inflammation of eyeball)

tendinous—*see* tenderness

tendonitis—*see* tendinitis

tenonitis—*see* tendinitis

tenser (more rigid; more tense) • **tensor** (a stretched muscle) • **tensure** (tension; stretching)

tensor—*see* tenser

tensure—*see* tenser

tentinous—*see* tenderness

tere—*see* tear

teres—*see* tears

terpene (unsaturated hydrocarbon) • **terpin** (antiseptic liquid)

terpin—*see* terpene

testes (pl. of *testis*) • **testis** (male reproductive gland) • **tests** (trials; examinations)

testis—*see* testes

tests—*see* testes

tetanic (relating to tetenus) • **titanic** (a chemical compound)

thermophilic (preferring heat) • **thermophylic** (resisting heat)

thermophylic—*see* thermophilic

thiamin or **thiamine** (a vitamin) • **thymin** (hormone of the thymus) •

thymine (a principal component of DNA) • **thymion** (wart)

thiamine—*see* thiamin

thio- (prefix showing sulfur replacement in a related compound) • **thiol** (analogue of *alcohol*)

thiol—*see* thio-

throe (a painful spasm) • **throw** (to discharge; to hurl)

throw—*see* throe

thymin—*see* thiamin

thymine—*see* thiamin

thymion—*see* thiamin

thyroid (endocrine gland) • **tyroid** (cheesy)

tic (a twitching; a sudden spasm) • **tick** (bloodsucking arachnid)

tick—*see* tic

tide (alternate rise and fall) • **tied** (closed off; fastened)

tied—*see* tide

tiers—*see* tears

tine (dentist's instrument) • **tinea** (ringworm)

tinea—*see* tine

titanic—*see* tetanic

toe (digit of the foot) • **tow** (flax in surgical dressing)

tow—*see* toe

trachelotomy (uterine incision) • **tracheotomy** (tracheal incision)

tracheotomy—*see* trachelotomy

tracked (followed a path) • **tract** (number of nerve fibers or organs)

tract—*see* tracked

trail (a track; record; consequence) •
trial (test, as of a drug)

trance (partly suspended animation) •
trans (relating to an arrangement
of genes) • trans- (prefix meaning
through or *across*)

trans—*see* trance

trans-—*see* trance

transamination (reaction involving
amino group) • transanimation
(reviving stillborn infant)

transanimation—*see* transamination

transposition (removal from one side
to another; metathesis) •
transposon (DNA segment)

transposon—*see* transposition

treacle (a medicinal compound used
in the treatment of poison) •
trickle (to fall in drops; to flow
slowly)

trephine (surgical saw) • trephone
(build-up of protoplasm)

trephone—*see* trephine

trial—*see* trail

trickle—*see* treacle

trochlea (pulley-like structure) •
trochlear (relating to trochlea or
to a muscle of the eye)

trochlear—*see* trochlea

trophic (relating to a mutation) •
tropic (relating to tropism;
influencing the action of a gland)

tropic—*see* trophic

tuba (tube or canal) • tubal (re: a
tube, especially the Fallopian tube)
• tuber (local swelling)

tubal—*see* tuba

tuber—*see* tuba

tubes (canals) • tubus (canal)

tubus—*see* tubes

tussal (relating to a cough) • tussle
(to fight; to struggle)

tussle—*see* tussal

tympanites (abdominal distention) •
tympanitis (middle ear
inflammation)

tympanitis—*see* tympanites

tyroid—*see* thyroid

U

ulna (large bone in forearm) • ulnar
(pertaining to the ulna or its
constituents)

ulnar—*see* ulna

unable—*see* enable

uncal (relating to the uncus) • uncle
(brother of one's father or mother)

uncle—*see* uncal

ungual (pertaining to the nails) •
ungula (extracting instrument)

ungula—*see* ungual

unique—*see* eunuch

uranyl (forms salts with acids) •
urinal (vessel for urine)

ureter (a canal carrying urine from
the kidney to the bladder) •
urethra (canal to discharge urine)

urethra—*see* ureter

urinal—*see* uranyl

uvea (middle coat of eye) • **uveal**
(pertaining to the uvea)

uveal—*see* uvea

uvula (soft palate projection) •
uvular (pertaining to the uvula)

uvular—*see* uvula

V

vaccine (preparation to produce
immunity) • **vaccinee** (a person
who has received a vaccine)

vaccinee—*see* vaccine

Valium (diazepam; tranquilizer) •
vallum (round, raised ridge)

vallum—*see* Valium

valva (flaps preventing reflux) •
valve (fold of membrane)

valve—*see* valva

valvula (small valve) • **valvulae** (pl.
of *valvula*) • **valvular** (pertaining
to a valve)

valvulae—*see* valvula

valvular—*see* valvula

variance (state of being different) •
variants (mutations)

variants—*see* variance

vas (a vessel; duct) • **vast** (large)

vasal (relating to a vas or vessel) •
vessel (a tube or canal)

vast—*see* vas

vector (a carrier of disease) • **victor**
(the winner in a struggle)

vena (vessel carrying blood to heart)
• **venae** (veins; pl. of *vena*)

venae—*see* vena

venous (relating to veins) • **venus**
(intercourse)

venular (about venules) • **venule**
(small vein; capillary vein)

venule—*see* venular

venus—*see* venous

vergence (inclining, as of eyeballs) •
virgins (people who never
experienced intercourse;
uncontaminated items)

vertex (crown; top of the head) •
vortex (to mix rapidly)

vertical (perpendicular; of the crown
of the head) • **verticil** (whorl)

verticil—*see* vertical

vesica (a bladder) • **vesicula** (a tiny
bladder) • **vesicular** (pertaining to
small sacs or bladders)

vesical (pertaining to bladder) •
vesicle (a small bladder)

vesicle—*see* vesical

vesicula—*see* vesica

vesicular—*see* vesica

vessel—*see* vasal

vial (a closed vessel, especially for
liquids) • **vile** (offensive;
disgusting; cheap)

vibrio (one member of genus *Vibrio*)
• *Vibrio* (genus of short, rod-
shaped organisms)

Vibrio—*see* vibrio

vice (defect in pathology; harmful habit) • vise (gripping tool)

victor—*see* vector

vile—*see* vial

villose or villous (having minute projections) • villus (minute projection of a mucous membrane)

villous—*see* villose

villus—*see* villose

viral (caused by virus) • virile (with masculine traits)

virgins—*see* vergence

virile—*see* viral

virose or virous (having poisonous qualities) • virus (a parasitic organism)

virous—*see* virose

virus—*see* virose

viscous (glutinous) • viscus (enclosed organs)

viscus—*see* viscous

vise—*see* vice

vitellin (protein in egg yolk) • vitelline (related to the egg yolk)

vitelline—*see* vitellin

vola (concave or hollow surface) • volar (palmar; plantar)

volar—*see* vola

vortex—*see* vertex

vulva (external female genital organs) • vulvar (pertaining to the vulva)

vulvar—*see* vulva

W

waist (narrow part of body above hips) • waste (to grow thin; excrement)

wait (to delay; to await) • weight (measure of body's pull by gravity)

ward (large hospital room) • wart (a horny skin elevation)

wart—*see* ward

waste—*see* waist

way (method, path) • weigh (to determine weight in pounds, grams, etc.) • whey (milk serum)

weak (lacking in strength; feeble) • week (seven consecutive days)

week—*see* weak

weigh—*see* way

weight—*see* wait

wen (a cyst) • when (at what time)

wheal (edema of the skin) • wheel (circular frame for turning)

wheel—*see* wheal

when—*see* wen

whey—*see* way

whole—*see* hole

write—*see* right

X-Y-Z

xanthene (crystal substance used in dyes) • **xanthine** (nitrogenous compound)

xanthine—*see* xanthene

xero- (combining form meaning *pertaining to dryness*) • **zero** (mathematical symbol) • **zero-** (combining form meaning *nothing* [0]; a starting point)

yoke (a device for joining together; to join together) • **yolk** (food stored in the ovum)

yolk—*see* yoke

zero—*see* xero-

zero-—*see* xero-

SECTION 3

Quick List of Correct Spellings

A

AASECT
ab-
ABC powder
abdomen
abdominal cavity
abducens nerve
abduct
abductor**
aberrant
aberration
abiogenesis
ablatio**
ablation**
-able
abled
abnormal behavior
abnormality
abnormal psychology
abortifacient
abortin**
abortion**
ABO system
abradant
abrasion
abrasive
abruptio
abscess
abscission
absolute
absorb**
absorption
absorptive state
abstinence
abulia
abuse
acacia**
Acacia**
acapnia**
acapnial**
acarid**
acathexia**
acathexis**
accident
accidentally
accommodation
Accutane

ACE bandage
A cells
ACE mixture
acentric
acephalic
acetabulum
acetal**
acetaminophen
acetanilide
acetic
acetophenetidin
acetyl**
acetylcholine
acetylsalicylic acid
achondroplasia
acid**
acid-fast bacteria
acidosis
acinus
acne
aconite
acorea**
acoria**
acoustic nerve
acquired
acquired immune deficiency
   syndrome
acr-
acrid**
acro-
acromegaly
ACTH
actin
acting out
Actinobacillus
Actinomyces bovis
actinomycin
actinomycosis
actinotherapy
action potential
active birth
active hyperemia
active immunity
active site
active transport
acupressure

acupuncture
acute
acute abdomen
acute brain disorders
acyclic
acyclovir
Adam's apple
adaptation
addict
addiction
addictive
Addison's disease
additive**
additive-free
adduct
adductor**
adenine
adenitis
adeno-
adenocarcinoma
adenoido-
adenoids
adenoma
adenosine
adenosine diphosphate
adenosine triphosphate
ADH
adherent
adhesion
adhesive compress
adhesive tape
adip-
adipic acid
adipo-
adipocyte
adipose
adjunctive chemotherapy
adjuvant therapy
Adler
Adlerian psychotherapy
adnexa
adnexa uteri
adnexitis
ADP
adrenal cortical hyperfunction
adrenal gland
adrenal hypofunction
adrenalin

adrenergic
adrenocorticotropic hormone
adrenosterone
adrenotrophin
adsorb**
adult
adverse event
aero-
aerobic
aerobics
aerocele**
aeroembolism
aerogenous**
aerophagia
aerosol**
aerosol therapy
aerotherapeutics
aerotherapy
afebrile
affect**
affective disorder
affective slumber
afferent**
afferent neuron
afferent pathway
affliction
affluemna
affluent**
afterbirth
agar**
agger**
agglutination
agglutinin
aggression
aggressive
agita
agnosia
agonal
agonist
agranular endoplasmic reticulum
agranulocytes
agranulocytosis
agraphia
ague
aides**
aids**
AIDS**
AIDS-related complex

AIDS test
AIDS victim
ailing
ailment**
air hunger
airsickness
alangine**
alanine**
Al-Anon**
alantin**
albinism
albumen**
albumin**
albumin-**
albumino-
albuminoid
albuminuria
alcohol
Alcoholics Anonymous
alcoholism
aldose
aldosterone
Alexander technique
alexia
-algia
algo-
alibido
alienation
aliment**
alimentary**
alimentary canal
alimentotherapy
alkalosis
Alka Seltzer
all-
allele
Allen-Doisy hormone
Allergan**
allergen**
allergist
allergy
allo-
allogenic
allograft
allopath**
allopathy**
all or none response
allosome

allosteric enzyme
allotrophic**
allotropic**
aloes
alopecia
alpha-amylase
alpha cells
alpha-fetoprotein
alpha rhythm
alpha wave
alternative medicine
altitude sickness
altrose
alveolar bone
alveolar pressure
alveolar ventilation
alveolo-
alveolus
Alzheimer's disease
AMA
amandin
amaurosis
ambivert
amblyo-
amblyopia
ambulance
ambulatory
ameba
amebiasis
amebic dysentery
ameleia**
amelia**
amenorrhea
amentia
American Medical Association
amidase
amidin**
amidine**
amino acid
aminopeptidase
aminopolypeptidase
aminopurine**
aminopyrine**
amitriptyline
ammonia
ammonium carbonate
ammonium chloride
amnesia

amnestic syndrome
amni-
amnio-
amniocentesis
amniography
amnioinfusion
amnion
amniotensin
Amniotin
amobarbital
amobarbital sodium
amoeba
amorphous**
amorphus**
amoxicillin
amphetamine
amphetamine sulfate
amphotericin
ampicillin
ampul**
ampule**
ampulla**
amputation
amyl-
amylase
amyl nitrite
amylo-
amylopectin
amylopsin
amyotrophic lateral sclerosis
Amytal
an-
ana-
anabolic steroid
anabolic steroid hormones
anabolism
Anacin
anaclasis**
anaclisis**
anacusis
anaerobic
anal**
analgesia
analgesic
analogues
anal personality
analyses**
analysis**

analytic psychology
analyzes**
anancastic personality
anankastic personality
anaphase
anaphylaxis
anatomy
anchyl/o-
androgen
androgenous**
androgynous**
androsterone
anemia
anencephaly
anesthesia
anesthesiologist
anesthesiology
anesthetic
anesthetist
aneuploidy
aneurism
angary macrophage
anger**
angi-
angina
angina pectoris
angio-
angiocardiography
angiography
angiohypertonia**
angiohypotonia**
angioma
angioplasty
angor**
anhydro-
anima**
animal**
animality
animus**
anise**
ankle
ankylosis
anlage
annulary
annulose**
annulus**
ano-
anodyne

anol**
anomalies
anomalous
anomia**
anomie**
anomous**
anorchous**
anorchus**
anorectal disorders
anorexia nervosa
anovulation
anoxia
ant-
Antabuse
antacid
antagonism
antagonist
ante**
ante-
antedate**
anteflexion
antegrade
antemortem
antenatel
antepartum
anterior
anterior chamber
anterior lobe disorder
anth-
anthelmintic
anthrax
anti**
anti-
antianxiety drug
antiarrhythmic
antibiotic
antibody
antibody negative
antibody positive
antibody seronegativity
antibody seropositivity
anticholinergic
anticipation
anticlotting
anticoagulant
anticonvulsant
antidepressant
antidiuretic

antidiuretic hormone
antidote**
antiemetic
antiflatulent
antifungal
antigen
antihistamine
anti-inflammatory
antimer**
antimere**
antimicin A
antimicrobial
antioxidant
antiprostaglandinsisobutyl nitrate
antipruritic
antipsychotics
antipyrine
antipyretic
antiseptic
antiserum
antishock trousers
antisocial personality
antispasmodic
antitoxin
antitussive
antivenin
antivirus
antrum
anulus**
anus**
anxiety
anxiety disorder
anxiety neurosis
anxiety reaction
aortitis
aort-
aorta
aortic arch
aortic-body chemoreceptor
aortic valve disease
aorto-
apatite**
apex
Apgar score
aphagia**
aphakia**
aphasia**
aphrodisia**

aphrodisiac**
aplastic anemia
apnea
apocrine
apocrine secretion
apoenzyme
apoplexy
apothecary
appendectomy
appendicitis
appendico-
appendix
appendo-
appetite**
appetite suppressant
application
applied psychology
apraxia
aqua-aerobics
aqueous
aqueous liquor
araban**
arabin**
arabinose
arachnoid villus
arbovirus
arc
ARC
arc-eye
archetyper
arcuate
arcuate vessels
arenavirus
arginase
arginine
Argyrol
arhythmia**
armamentarium
armpit
arnica
aromatherapy
aromatic spirits of ammonia
arousal
arrhythmia**
arsenic
arsenotherapy
arterial baroreceptors
arterio-

arteriolar resistance
arteriole
arteriolo-
arteriosclerosis
arteritis**
artery
arthritis**
arthro-
arthroscope
arthroscopy
artificial
artificial heart
artificial insemination
artificial kidney
artificial limb
artificial lung
asbestos**
asbestosis**
ascending colon
ascorbic acid
-ase
asepsis
asexual
asitia
aspartic acid
aspect
asphyxiation
aspiration
aspirator
aspirin
assessment
assimilation
asthenic reaction
asthma
astigmatism
astragaloid
astringent
asylum
asymptomatic
asymptomaticity
Atabrine
atavism
ataxia
atelo-
athero-
atheroma
atherosclerosis
athlete's foot

atlas
atom
atomic**
atonic**
atony
atopy
ATP
atresia
atrium
atrophy
atropine
attendant
attending
attending physician
attenuated virus
attrition
audiogram
audiology
audiometer
auditive**
auditory cells
augmentation mammoplasty
aura**
aural**
Aureomycin
auricle
auscultation
autism
autoclave
autoclaving
autogenic training
autograft
autoimmune
autoimmune disease
autologous

automaticity
automatin**
automation**
automaton**
autonomic
autopsy
autoregulation
autoserum therapy
autosomal recessive
autosome
auxiliary**
average length of stay
aversion therapy
Avertin
avoid**
avoidance reaction
avoidant personality
avulsion
axial
axilla
axillary**
axillary dissection
axillary hair
axiom**
axion**
axis
axogenous**
axon**
axone**
axon transport
azaserine
azidothymadine
azoospermia
AZT

B

Babinski
baby-battering
BAC
Bachman**
Bachmann*
bacill-
bacillary dysentery
bacilli**

bacillin**
bacillus
bacitracin
back
backache
backbone
backup hospital
bacteremia

bacteri-
bacteria
bacterial
bacterial endocarditis
bacterial therapy
bactericide**
bacteriocidin**
bacteriocin**
bacteriology
bacteriolysins
bacteriophage**
bacteriophagia**
bacteriostat
bacteriotherapy
bacteriotropic**
bacteriotropin**
bacterium
bacteroid**
*Bacteroides***
bad breath
Baelz**
Baer**
Baeyer**
baking soda
balance**
balanitis
bald**
baldness
ball**
Ballance**
ball-and-socket joint
balloon
balloon angioplasty
ballottement
balm**
Balme**
balm of Gilead
balsam
bamboo spine
bamboo sugar
bandage
Band Aid
band-aid sterilization
Banting
bar**
Bar**
barbital
barbiturate

barbituric acid
baric
barium enema
barium meal
barium sulfate
barley sugar
Barlow's syndrome
baroreceptor
Barr body
barren
barrier contraceptives
Bartholin glands
Barton bandage
basal**
basal body temperature method
basal-cell carcinoma
basal ganglia
basal metabolic rate
basal metabolism
base
based**
basement membrane
bases**
basic
basil**
basis**
Basle Nomina Anatomica
basophil
bast**
bath**
bathe**
batter
battle fatigue
bawl**
Bayle's**
B cell
bed occupancy
bedpan
bed rest
bedridden
bedside manner
bedsore
bedwetting
beet sugar
behavior
behavioral medicine
behaviorism
behavior therapy

bel**
belch
belie**
Bell**
belladonna
belle indifference
Bell's palsy
belly**
bellybutton
bends
benign
benign orgasmic headaches
Benzadrine
benzene**
benzin**
benzine**
benzocaine
benzoin**
benzoyl**
benzyl**
beriberi
berth**
bestiality
beta**
Beta**
beta-amylase
beta blocker
beta cells
beta rhythm
beta wave
better**
bhang
bi-
Bial**
bias**
bibliotherapy
bicarbonate of soda
biceps
bichloride of mercury
bicuspid
bidet
bifocal
bifurcation
bile**
bile duct
bile salts
bili-
biliary colic

bilious
bilirubin
bilirubinemia
Billig exercises
Billings method
binder boric acid
binding site
Binet
binge-purge syndrome
bioassay
bioenergetics
bioethics
biofeedback
biological clock
biologics
bioluminescence
biomedicine
bionics
biopsy
bios*
biose**
biosis**
biosynthesis
biotech**
biotechnology
biotherapy
biotic**
biotin
bipolar disorder
birth**
birth canal
birth control pill
birth defect
birthmark
bismuth
bistoury
bisulfate**
bisulfide**
bisulfite**
bite-wing radiograph
black-and-blue mark
black eye
blackheads
black lung
blackout**
black out**
blackwater fever
bladder

bladder augmentation
blank-state hypothesis
blast-
-blast
blasto-
Blastomyces brasiliensis
blastomycosis
bleaching powder
bleb
bleeder
blennorrhagia
bleomycin
blephar-
blepharitis
blepharo-
blepharoplasty
blindness
blister
bloc**
Bloch**
block**
blocker
block grants
blocking
blocking antibody
Blocq**
blood
blood alcohol concentration
blood alcohol content
blood bank
blood-brain barrier
blood clot
blood component
blood count
blood donor
blood group
bloodletting
bloodmobile
blood poisoning
blood pressure
blood pressure cuff
bloodstream
blood sugar
blood types
blood typing
blood urea nitrogen
bloody flux

blotch
blow
blue baby
Blue Cross
blue ointment
Blue Shield
blurred vision
B lymphocyte
BMR
board certified physician
boarder baby
body
bodybuilding
body contouring
body fluids
body language
body mechanics
body scanner
body schema
body wrap
boil
bolus
bond
bone
bone graft
bony
booster shot
borax
borborygmus
borderline
borderline personality
Bordetella
Borelia
boric acid
born**
borne**
Bornholm disease
Borrelia
bosom
boss
botulin
botulism
bouba
bougie
bowel**
bowel evacuant
bowl**

brace
braces
brachial
brachial nerve
brachy-
brady-
bradycardia
bradykinin
bradyphagia**
bradyphasia**
brain
brain damage
brain stem
brake**
breach**
breadth**
break**
breakout**
break out**
breakthrough bleeding
break wind
breast
breast augmentation
breastbone
breast-feed
breast ptosis
breast reduction
breath**
Breathalyzer
breathe**
breathing
breathlessness
breech**
breech presentation
bridge
bright**
Bright**
Bright's disease
Brioschi
Bristol-Myers Squibb
British gum
broach
broad-spectrum
bromide
bromidrosis
bromine
Bromo Seltzer

bronch-
bronchi-
bronchial**
bronchial asthma
bronchio-
bronchiole**
bronchitis
bronchodilator
bronchoscope
bronchospasm
bronchus
brow
brown lung
brucella
brucellosis
bruise
bruiser
bruit
bruxism
buba**
bubo**
bubonic plague
buccal cavity
bucco-
bucktooth
bud**
Budd**
buffered aspirin
Bufferin
buffer therapy
bulbous**
bulb syringe
bulbus**
bulimia
bulk flow
bulla
bump
BUN
bunion
burn
burnout
Burow's solution
Burroughs-Wellcome
bursa
bursitis
burso-
butacaine

161

butacaine sulfate
buts**
buttocks
butts**

butyl
butyrophenone
bypass
byssinosis

C

cachet
cachexia
caco-
cacodontia
cadaver
caffeine
caisson disease
calamine lotion
calc-
calcaneus
calci-
calcine**
calcinosis
calcitonin
calcium
calcium carbonate
calcium channel blocker
calculous**
calculus**
calendar method
calendar rhythm
calf
calibrate
calicine**
caliculus**
calisthenics
calix**
call**
callose**
callous**
callus**
calmodulin
calomel
calor**
calx**
calyx**
camera
cAMP
camphor**

Campylobacter
canal
cancer**
cancrum
*Candida***
Candida albicans
candidal vaginitis
candidiasis
candidid**
candy striper
cane sugar
canine
canker**
cannabis
cannabism**
cannibalism**
cannula
cannulation
cantharides
capelet**
capillary
capillary network
capita**
capital**
capitate
capitation**
caplet**
caproin**
caprone**
capsid
capsula**
capsule**
captation**
caput
carate**
carbohydrase
carbohydrate
carbolic acid
carbomycin

carbon
carbonic anhydrase
carboxypeptidase
carbuncle**
carcino-
carcinogen
carcinoma
cardi-
-cardia**
cardiac**
cardiac arrest
cardiac hormone
cardiac massage
cardiac muscle
cardiac output
cardiac stenosis
cardio-
cardiograph
cardiography
cardioid**
cardiology
cardiomyopathy
cardiopulmonary resuscitation
cardiorespiratory endurance
Cardio salsa
cardioscope
cardiotherapy
carditis
career**
care-giver
carer**
caries**
carina
carnitine
carotene
carotid**
carotid artery
carotid-body chemoreceptor
carpal
carpal tunnel syndrome
carpus
carrier**
carries**
carrot**
carsickness
cartilage
caruncle**
cascara

cascara sagrada
case
case history
casein
caseinogen
cassolette
cast
castor oil
castration
cat-
cata-
catabolism
catalepsy
catamenia
cataphora**
cataphoria**
cataplexy
cataract
catarrh
catastrophic coverage
catatonia
catchment area
catecholamines
cath-
catharsis
cathartic
catheter
catheterization
catholicon
CAT scan
cat-scratch disease
caud-
cauda**
cauda equina
caudo-
caul**
cauliflower ear
causal agent
caustic
cauter**
cauterize
cava**
cave**
cavernous
cavity
cavum
cec-
cecal

ceco-
cecum
-cele**
celiac disease
cell**
-cell
cell division
cell-mediated immunity
cellobiose
cells
cellulite reduction
cellulitis
cellulose
cementum
censor**
census**
Centers for Disease Control
-centesis
central hearing loss
central nervous system
central thermoreceptors
centrifuge
centrioles
centromere
centrum
cephalalgia
cephalgia
cephalo-
cephaloridine
cerated**
cereal**
cerebellum**
cerebral
cerebral aqueduct
cerebral cortex
cerebral cranials
cerebral hemorrhage
cerebral palsy
cerebro-
cerebrospinal fever
cerebrospinal fluid
cerebrospinal system
cerebrovascular accident
cerebrum**
cereous**
Cereus**
cerous**
cerumen**

cerumenolytic
cervic-
cervical cap
cervical dysplasia
cervical erosion
cervical incompetence
cervical-mucus method
cervical nerve
cervical os
cervical vertebrae
cervicectomy
cervici-
cervicitis
cervix
Cesarean section
cessation
CG
cGMP
chaining
chalasia**
chalaza**
chamfer**
chancre**
chancroid
change of life
channel
chapping
character disorder
Charcot
Charcot's joint
charge nurse
charity patient
charley horse
chart**
charta**
checkup
cheek
cheekbone
cheil-
cheilitis
cheilo-
cheiloplasty
cheilosis
chelating agents
chem-
chemi-
chemical dependency
chemical peel

chemical sense
chemical specificity
chemical stimulation of the brain
chemist
chemo-
chemoreceptors
chemoresistance
chemosynthesis
chemotaxis
chemotherapy
chest
chest x-ray
Cheyne-Stokes respiration
chickenpox
chief cells
chief resident
chilblain
child
child abuse
childbed fever
child development
children's hospital
chilo-
chin
chip
chir-
chiro-
chiropodist
chiropody
chiropractic
chiropractic adjustment
chiropractor
chirurgical
chlamydia
chlor-
chloral
chloral hydrate
chloramine
chloramine-T
chloramphenicol
chlordiazepoxide
chlorine
chlorine of lime
chloro-
chloroform
Chloromycetin
chlorophenol**
chlorophyll

chloroplast
chloroquine
chlorphenol**
chlorpromazine
chlortetracycline
chocolate
choke
choking
chol-
cholangia
chole-
cholecyst
cholecystectomy
cholecystis**
cholecystitis**
cholecystokinin
cholelithiasis
cholera
choleraic**
choleric**
cholesterol
cholinergic
cholo-
chondr/i/o-
chondrotropic hormone
chorda
chorea
chorioidea
chorionic gonadotropin
choroid coat
choroid plexus
chromaprotein
chromat-
chromatid
chromatin
chromato-
chromium
chromosomal aberration
chromosome
chronic
chronic cystic mastitis
chronic fatigue syndrome
chrysotherapy
chyme
chymotrypsin
Ciba
cicatrix
cidal

165

cilia
ciliary body
cilium**
cin-
cine**
cino-
circle
circulatory system
circumcision
circumstance
cirrhosis
cirrus**
cite**
citrate of magnesia
citric acid cycle
claimant
clamp
claudication
claustrophobia
clavicle
clavicul/o-
clawfoot
clearance
cleft palate
client-centered psychotherapy
climacteric
climatotherapy
climax
clinic
clinical dextran
clinical medicine
clinical psychology
clinical thermometer
clip
clitoridectomy
clitoris
clomiphene
clone
closed circulatory system
closed panel practice
clostridium
clot
clove oil
cloxacillin
clubbing
clubfoot
clupeine
cluster headache

CNS
coagulated protein
coagulation
coal tar
coat
cobalamin
cobalamine
cobalt
cobalt therapy
cocaine
cocainism
Coccidioides immitis
coccidioidomycosis
coccus**
*Coccus***
coccyg/o-
coccygeal nerve
coccyx
cochlea**
cochlear**
cochleare**
cochlear nerve
cocoa
code call
codeine
cod-liver oil
coenzyme
cofactor
coffee
cognitive psychology
cognitive service
co-insurance
coital
col-
cold
colds**
cold sore
cold therapy
coles**
Colgate-Hoyt
coli-
colic
colicky
colicky pain
colitis
collagen
collagen diseases
collagen injection

collagenolytic
collagen vascular disease
collapse
collapsed lung
collapse therapy
collar**
collarbone
Colles**
collodion
colloid
collum**
collyrium
colo-
colocynth
colon
colonic irrigation
colony
color**
color blindness
colorectal cancer
colostomy
colostomy bag
colp-
colpeurynter
colpitis
colpo-
colposcope
column**
coma
combat fatigue
comedo
command neuron
commissura
common cold
communicable
community hospital
community medicine
community psychology
compact**
compacta**
compact bone
compatible
compensation
compensatory growth
compensatory reaction
complement**
complementary medicine
complete blood count

complex
complex carbohydrate
compliance
complication
compliment**
composite
compound fracture
comprehensive medical insurance
compress
compressed air sickness
compromised host
compulsion
compulsive personality
computerized axial tomography
conceive
concentrate
concept
concha
concretion
concurrent therapy
condensation
condition
condom
conducting portion
conducting system
conductive hearing loss
condyle
condyloma
condylomata acuminata
cone
cone biopsy
confinement
confusion
congenital
congestion
congestive heart failure
conjectiva
conjoint therapy
conjugal
conjunctivitis
Connaught
connective tissue
connective tissue cells
connective tissue disorders
consanguinity
conscience**
conscious**
conservative treatment

constipation
constitutional psychology
constitutional therapy
constrictor
consultation
consulting psychology
consumption
contact**
contact dermatitis
contact therapy
contagious
contaminant
contamination
continent
contra-
contraceptive
contraceptive foam
contract**
contractility
contraction
contraction time
contraindicated
contraindication
contrast
contrecoup
control
control system
contusion
convalescent
convergence
convergence insufficiency
conversion disorder
conversion reaction
convulsion
coordination
co-payment
copper
copr-
copro-
coprolith
coprophilia
cor**
cord clamp
cordotomy
core**
core temperature
corn
cornea

corneal reflex
corneal transplant
corn sugar
cornu
corolla
corona
coronary**
coronary artery
coronary artery bypass
coronary artery bypass graft
coronary artery disease
coronary care unit
coronary heart disease
coronary infarction
coronary occlusion
coronary thrombosis
coroner**
corpse**
corpus**
corpus callosum
corpuscle
corpus luteum
corrective
correlation
cortex
cortical
cortico-
corticosterone
corticotropin
corticotropin releasing hormone
cortisol
cortisone
Corynebacterium
coryza
cosmetic surgery
cosmid
cost effectiveness
costo-
cotransport
cotton
cotton ball
cotton swab
couching
cough
cough syrup
Coumadin
counter
countercurrent multiplier system

168

counterirritant
countertransport
cowpox
coxa
CPR
crab louse
crack
cradle
cramp
crani-
cranial
cranial cavity
craniectomy
cranio-
craniograph
craniopathy
cranium
crapulent
creatine**
creatine phosphate
creatinine**
crenation
crepitation
crepitus
crescent
cresol
crest
cretinism
crib death
crick
cricoid cartilage
crippling
crisis
crista
critical
crook
cross-bridge
crossed eyes
cross-extensor reflex
crossing-over
crotch
croup
crown
crucial
crus**
crust**
crutch
cry-

cryo-
cryobank
cryobirth
cryocautery
cryonic suspension
cryosurgery
cryotherapy
crypt-
cryptic
crypto-
cryptococcosis
Cryptococcus neoformans
cryptogenic
crystallin**
crystalline**
C-section
cuboid
cuff
culdoscopy
cultural alienation
cultural relativism
culture
cumulative drugs
cuneiform
cunnilingus
curare
curative
cure
cure-all
curette
current
curvature of the spine
Cushing's disease
cusp
cuspid
cut
cutaneous
cuticle
cyano-
cyanosis
cyclazocine
cyclic AMP
cyclic GMP
cycloid
cyclopropane
cycloserine
cyclothyme
cyclothymic

cyclothymic personality
cyst
cyst-
cystectomy
cysti-
cystic duct
cystic fibrosis
cystine
cystitis
cysto-
cystography
cystoma
cystoscopy
cyt-
-cyte**

cyto-
cytochrome
cytogenetics
cytoglobulin
cytokinesis
cytology**
cytomegalovirus
cytoplasm
cytoprotective
cytoscope
cytosine
cytoskeleton
cytotoxin
cytotoxic T cells

D

D & C
dacry/o-
dactyl
dactyl-
dactylo- (pre)
dactylology
daily**
Dalkon shield
dally**
daltonism
dandruff
dark adaptation
Darvon
data
date sugar
days**
daze**
DC
DDS
DDSc
de-
dead**
dead space
deaf muteness
deafness
deaminase
death certificate

debility
debridement
decade**
decadent**
decayed**
decease**
decedent**
decent**
dechloridation**
dechlorination**
decidua**
deciduate**
deciduoma**
decision**
decompression
decompression sickness
decongestant
decrease**
decrees**
decrement**
decrepit
decubation
decubitus ulcer
deed**
defecation
defect
defense

defense mechanism
defer**
deference**
deferens**
defibrillator
deficiency disease
deficient**
deficit**
definite**
definitive**
deformation
deformity
defuse**
degeneration
degenerative
deglutition
degrease**
degrees**
dehiscence
dehydration
dehydrocorticosterone
deletion**
delimit
delirium
delirium tremens
deltoid
delude**
delusion**
delusional syndrome
dementia
dementians
dementia praecox
Demerol
demonology
demote**
demulcent
dendrite
dengue**
denial
denote**
dens**
dense**
dent-
dental
dental drill
dental extraction forceps
dental floss
dental hygienist

dental surgery
dental technician
dentes**
denti-
denticle
dentifrice
dentin
dentine
dentist
dentistry
dento-
dentofacial
dents**
dentures
deoxyhemoglobin
deoxyribonucleic acid
deoxyribose
dependence
dependency
dependent personality
depersonalization
depigmenting agent
depilatory
depolarization
Depo-Provera
deposition**
depressant
depression
depressive neurosis
depressive psychosis
depressive reaction
depth psychology
derm-
-derm
derma-
-derma
dermabrasion
dermal
dermal sheath
dermata-
-dermata
dermatitis**
dermato-
dermatology
dermatome
dermatophytosis
dermatosis**
dermatotherapy

-dermis
dermo-
dermoid cyst
dermostosis**
descendants**
descendens**
descending colon
descent**
Des daughter
desensitization
desiccant**
desiccate**
designer drug
desipramine
desm/o-
desmosome
desoxycorticosterone
desoxyephedrine
desperate**
DET
detached retina
deterioration
detoxification
detriment**
detritus
detumescence
developmental psychology
deviance
deviated septum
deviation
dexamethasone
Dexamyl
Dexedrine
dexterous**
dextran**
dextrin**
dextrinogenic enzyme
dextro-
dextroamphetamine sulfate
dextrose**
dextrous**
diabetes
diabetes insipidus
diabetes mellitus
diabetic**
diabetid**
diabetide**
Diabinese

diabrotic**
diaclasis**
diaclast**
diacritic**
diacritical**
diad**
diagnoses**
diagnosis**
diagnosis-related group
diagram**
Dial
dialysis
dialysis machine
diaper rash
diaphanoscope
diaphoresis
diaphragm**
diaphysis
diarrhea**
diarrhemia**
diastalsis**
diastase**
diastasis**
diastole
diastolic pressure
diathermy
diathermy knife
diathermy machine
diathesis
diathetic**
diazepam
dibenzoxazepines
dibucaine
Dick-Read
dicoumarin
dicromat**
dicromate**
dideoxyinosine
die**
died**
diet**
dietetic**
dietetics**
diethylstilbestrol
diethyltryptamine
dietician
dietotherapy
differ**

difference**
differential diagnosis
differently abled
diffuse**
diffusion
diffusion equilibrium
digestion
digestive system
digit
digitalin**
digitalis**
Digitalis**
digital nerve
digitoxin**
digoxin**
dihydrostreptomycin
diiodotyrosine
Dilantin
dilate**
dilatation**
dilation**
dilation and curettage
dilation and evacuation
dilute**
dilution**
dimethyltryptamine
diphenyldantoin
diphtheria**
diplegia
diplococci
diplococcus
*Diplodia***
diploic**
diploid**
diploidy**
diplomate
diplopia**
dips/o-
*Dipteria***
disability
disapprove**
disburse**
discharge
discission**
disclose
discreet**
discrete**
discus**

discuss**
disease**
disillusion**
disinfectant**
disinfestant**
disinhibition
disintegrate
dislocation
disorder
disorientation
disparate**
dispensary
disperse**
displaced aggression
displacement
disposition**
disprove**
dissect
dissociation reaction
dissociative disorder
dissolution**
dissolve
dist/o-
distal**
distemper
distill**
disulfuram
diuretic
diurnal**
diurnule**
divergence
diverticular disease
diverticulitis**
diverticulosis**
dizygotic twins
dizziness
do**
doctor
Doctor of Medicine
does**
dollar**
dolor**
dominant gene
dominant hemisphere
donee**
donor**
donor insemination
dopa**

dopamine
dope**
dors/o-
dorsal
dorsal dyspepsia
dose**
dose-response phenomenon
dosimetry
double helix
double vision
douching
dowager's hump
Down syndrome
Dr.
dracontiasis
drain
drain tube
Dramamine
dream
dressing
DRG
droplet infection
drops**
dropsy**
drug
druggist
duct
ductal**
ductile**
ductless gland
ductule**
ductus
ductus deferens
due**
duel innervation

duller**
dumping
dumping syndrome
dung**
duoden/o-
duodenal ulcer
duodenum
Du Pont
dura mater
dwarfism
dye**
dyed**
dye therapy
dys-
dyscheria**
dyscholia**
dyschroia**
dyschylia**
dyscoria**
dysentery
dysfunction
dyslalia
dyslexia
dysmenorrhea
dyspareunia
dyspepsia
dysphagia**
dysphasia**
dysplasia**
dyspnea
dystonic**
dystopic**
dystrophy
dysuria

E

-eal
ear
earache
ear canal
eardrum
earlobe
earwax
ebrious
ecchymosis

eccrine
eccrine gland
ecdemic**
echo
echocardiogram**
echocardiograph**
echocardiography**
echography**
echophrasia**

174

echopraxia**
eclampsia
eclectic psychology
ecphoria**
ect-
-ectasia
-ectasis
ecto-
ectocornea
ectoderm**
ectomorph**
-ectomy
ectopic focus
ectopic pregnancy
eczema
edema
-edema
edestin
EEG arousal
effacement
effect**
effector
efferent**
efferent neuron
efflorescence
effluent**
ego
egoism**
egotism**
Ehrlich
either**
ejaculate
EKG
elastic
elastic bandage
elastin
Elavil
elbow
electr-
Electra complex
electric
electrical stimulation of the brain
electro-
electrocardiogram**
electrocardiograph**
electrocardiography**
electrocardiophonogram
electrocautery

electrode
electroencephalograph
electrograph
electrokymograph**
electrolysis
electrolyte
electrometrogram**
electromyogram**
electromyograph**
electromyography**
electron
electrophoresis
electrosurgery
electrotherapy
electuary
elementary**
elephantiasis
elephantman's disease
Eli Lilly
ELISA
elixir
Elkins-Sinn
eluate**
elude**
elusive**
elute**
elution**
em-
emaciation
emanation
emasculation
embolism
embolus
embryo
embryology
emergency
emergency medical service
emergency medical technician
emergency room
emergency ward
-emesis
emetic
-emia
eminentia
emission**
emollient
emotion
emotional instability reaction

175

emphysema
empiric risk
Empirin
empyema
emulsification
en-
enable**
enamel
encephal/o-
-encephalia
encephalitis
encrust**
end/o-
end-diastolic volume
endemia**
endemic**
endermatic**
endermic**
endocarditis
endocrine gland
endocrine system
endocrinology
endocrinotherapy
endocytosis
endoderm**
endodontics**
endodontist**
endometrial carcinoma
endometriosis
endomorph**
endopeptidase
endoplasmic reticulum
endorphin
endoscope
endotracheal tube
endyma**
enema**
enervate**
enervation
engineering psychology
enhancement
enhancer
ent-
Entamoeba histolytica
enter/o-
enteritis
enterocele
enterocronin

enterogastrone
enterokinese
enterostomy
enteroviral diseases
entoderm**
enuresis
enzyme
enzyme induction
enzyme-linked immunosorbent
   assay
enzymology
eosinophil
ep/epi-
ephedrine
epicanthic fold
epicanthus
epidemic**
epidemiology
epidermis
epidermophyton
epidermophytosis
epididymis
epigastrium
epiglottis
epilepsy
epinephrine
epiphysis
episi/o-
episiotomy
episode
epistaxis
epithelial cells
epithelioma
epithelium
Epsom salts
Epstein-Barr syndrome
equal
Equanil
equilibrium potential
Erb's palsy
erect**
erectile dysfunction
erection**
erector
-ergic
ergot
ergotherapy
erogenous**

erotic**
erotica**
eroto-
eruct**
eructation**
erupt**
eruption
erysipelas
erythema**
erythro-
erythrocyte
erythrocyte sedimentation rate
erythromycin
erythropoiesis
erythropoietin
erythrose
escape
escapism
eschar**
escherichia
esophag/o-
esophageal orifice
esophagus
essential
essential amino acids
essential nutrients
esterase
esthesi/o-
estradiol
estrin
estriol
estrogen
estrone
estrous**
estrus**
ether**
ethmoid
ethnology**
ethology**
ethyl
ethyl chloride
ethylene
ethylene oxide
etio-
etiology
eu-
eucalyptus
eukaryote

eunuch**
eunuchoidism
euphoria**
eustachian tube
euthanasia
evacuation
evacuator
evaluation
everyday**
every day**
everyone**
every one**
everything**
every thing**
evulsion
ex/o-
examination
examine
examining room
exanthematous
Excedrin
exchange transfusion
excision
excitability
excitation
excitatory synapse
excite
excrement
excretion
exercise**
exhalation
exhibitionism
existential neurosis
existential psychotherapy
exocrine gland
exocytosis
exodontics
exodontist
exogenous**
exon**
exophthalmic goiter
exorcise**
exotic**
expanders
expectant
expectorant
experiment
experimental psychology

expert
expiration
expiratory reserve volume
explode
exploratory surgery
explosion
expressivity
expulsion
extenders
extension
extensor
exterior
external
external cuneiform
extra-
extracellular fluid

extract
extraction
extrahepatic
extremitas
extremity
extrinsic clotting pathway
extrovert
eye
eyeball
eyebrow
eyed**
eyelash
eyelid
eye socket
eye tuck
eyewash

F

face
facelift
facet**
facial**
facial nerve
facies**
facilitated diffusion
facilitation
facility
faction**
factitious disorders
factor
factor eight
factor VIII
facts**
faculty
Fahrenheit
failure
faint**
fainting
fair**
faith healer
fallopian tube
fallout**
fall out**
falls**
false**

false labor
false pregnancy
false rib
false teeth
falx**
family
family doctor
family medicine
family practitioner
fantasy
fare**
farsightedness
fascia**
fascial**
fascia lata
fascicle**
fasciculi
fastidious
fastigium
fat
fatal**
fatigue
fatty acids
fatty liver
fauces**
faucet**
favus

fax**
fear
feat**
febri-
febrifuge
febrile**
fecal softeners
feces**
fecund
feeble**
feedback
feet**
feint**
fellatio
female
feminine
feminine hygiene
femor/o-
femoral nerve
femur
fenestration
fennel**
feral**
ferment**
fermentation
ferning
ferritin
ferrous
ferrule**
fertile days
fertility drug
fertilize
fester
fet/o-
fetal**
fetal alcohol syndrome
fetal distress
fetish
fetishism
fetus
fever
fever blister
fever therapy
fiber
fibrae
fibril**
fibrillation
fibrin

fibrinogen
fibrinolytic
fibro-
fibroadenoma
fibrocystic breast
fibrocystic disease
fibroepithelial tumor
fibroids
fibroma
fibrosarcoma
fibrose**
fibrosis
fibrous**
fibul/o-
fibula
fight-or-flight response
figure-of-eight
fila**
filament
filar**
filariasis
file**
filing**
fill**
filling**
filtration
filum**
filum terminate
finger
finger bones
first aid
first-degree burn
fiscal**
fission
fissura**
fissure**
fist
fists**
fistula
fit
fits**
fixation
fixed-fee
flashburn
flagella
Flagyl
flammable
flap

flat
flattened effect
flatulence
flatus
flavin**
flavine**
flavone**
fleas**
flecks**
fleece**
flees**
flesh
flew**
flex**
flexion
flexion reflex
flexor**
flexor muscle
flexura**
flexure**
flicker
flight of ideas
flight reaction
floater
floating rib
flocks**
flocs**
floor**
flow
flu**
fluctuate
fluid
fluor**
fluorane**
fluorene**
fluorine**
fluoroscope
fluoroscopy
flush
flux**
foam
focus
Foley catheter
folic acid
Folin
folk medicine
follicle
follicle-stimulating hormone

follow-up
foment**
food poisoning
fool**
for**
foramen
forceps
forces**
fore**
fore-**
forearm
forehead
foreign
forensic medicine
foreplay
formaldehyde
formalin
formative
fornix
for-profit
forth**
fossa
foul
four**
fourchette
fourth**
fovea centralis
fraction**
fracture
fracture reduction
fradicin
fragile
frambesia
frays**
free radical
frees**
freeze**
Freud
freudian psychoanalysis
friable mass
friction
frigid
frigidity
frigotherapy
frontal
frontal lobe
frostbite
frozen section

frozen shoulder
fructose
fruit sugar
frustrated
fucose**
*Fucus***
fuel**
-fuge
*Fugu***
fugue**
full**
full-blown AIDS
functional disorder

functionalism
fundus
fungal infections
fungicides
fungus
funiculus
furfural**
furfurol**
furfuryl**
furuncle
furunculus
fusion

G

GABA
gait
galact-
galactan**
galactans**
galactase**
galacto-
galactophagous**
galactophygous**
galactose**
galactosemia
galactotherapy
galea**
galena**
gall
gallbladder
gallein**
gallin**
gallon**
gallstone
gamete
gamete intra-fallopian transfer
gamma-aminobutyric acid
gamma globulin
ganglia
ganglion
gangrene
ganja
Ganser's syndrome

Gantrism
gap junction
gargle
gas
gaseous
gash
gastr/o-
gastrectomy
gastric juice
gastric lavage
gastric ulcer
gastrin
gastritis
gastrocele**
gastrocnemius
gastrocoele**
gastroenteritis
gastroenterology
gastrointestinal tract
gastroscope
gatekeeper
Gaucher
Gaucher's disease
*Gaultheria***
gaultherin**
gauze**
gaze**
Geiger
Geigy

gel
gelatinous
gel-filled implant
gelose**
gelosis**
gen/o-
gender
gender dysphoria
gene
gene frequency
Genentech
gene pool
general
general anesthetic
general medicine
general practitioner
generic
generic-name drug
genesial stage
genesis
-genesis
gene therapy
genetic
-genetic
genetic code
genetic counseling
genetic engineering
genial**
-genic
genit/o-
genital**
genital herpes
genitals
genital warts
genitourinary
genius**
genome
genomic DNA
genotype
gentian violet
genu**
genus**
ger/o-
geranial**
geraniol**
geriatrics**
geriatrist**
germ

German measles
germicidal lamp
germicidal soap
germicide
geront/o-
gerontology
gestalt
gestation
gestosis
GFR
gibbous**
gibbus**
GIFT
gigantism
gingiv/o-
gingiva
gingivitis
GI series
gladiolus
gland
glands**
glandula**
glandular**
glandular fever
glandular system
glandular therapy
glans**
Glauber's salt
glaucoma
gliadin
glial cells
gliding joint
glioma
globi**
globin**
globulin
glomerul/o-
glomerular filtration rate
glomerulonephritis
gloss-
glossitis
glosso-
glossopalatine arch
glossopharyngeal nerve
glottis
glucagon
glucase**
glucocorticoid

gluconeogenesis
glucose**
glucose tolerance test
glutamic acid
glutaminase
glutaraldehyde
gluten**
glutenin
gluteus
glutin**
glyc-
glycerin
glycerite
glycerogel
glycerogelatin
glycerol
glycine**
Glycine**
glyco-
glycogen
glycogenesis**
glycogenolysis
glycogenosis**
glycolipid
glycolysis
glycolytic fast fibers
glycoprotein
glycos-
glycoso-
glycosuria
-gnathus
gnosia**
goiter
gold therapy
Golgi apparatus
Golgi tendon organs
gomer
gon-
gonad
gonadotropin
gonadotropin releasing hormone
gonial**
gonidial**
gonion**
gonium**
gono-
gonococcal urethritis
gonococcus

gonorrhea
goose bumps
goose flesh
gout
GP
graafian follicle
Grafenberg spot
graft**
gram**
Gram**
-gram
gram/o-
gramicidin
gram-negative bacteria
gram-positive bacteria
grand mal
granula**
granular**
granular endoplasmic reticulum
granule**
granulocyte
granuloma
grape sugar
-graph
graphed**
-graphy
Graves' disease
gravid**
gravida**
gravidity**
gravity**
gray market
gray matter
greater curvature
grip**
gripe**
grippe**
griseofulvin
groin
ground substance
group insurance
group practice
growth
growth hormone
gtt
guaiac test
guanine
Guillain-Barré

guilt
gullet
gulose
gum
gurney
gut**
gutta**
gutter**
Guttmacher Institute

guttur**
gynec-
gyneco-
gynecologist
gynecology
gyrosa**
gyrose**
gyrus**

H

habit**
habitat**
habitual**
habituate**
hacking
hair
hair follicle
hairy**
half**
half-life
halitosis
hallucinate
hallucination
hallucinogen
hallux
halocaine
halve**
halves**
hamartoma**
hamate
hammertoe
hamstring
hamulus**
hand
handicap
handicapped
hangnail
hangover
hang-up**
hang up**
Hansen**
Hansen's disease
Hanson**

haploid
haploidy
hard**
hard of hearing
hard palate
harelip
harry**
hashish
haunch**
have**
Haversian canals
hay fever
head**
headache
headache powder
heal**
healer
health administrator
Health Care Financing Adminis-
    tration
health facility
health insurance
health maintenance organization
hear**
heart**
heart attack
heartbeat
heartburn
heart defects
heart failure
heart-lung machine
heart murmur
heat exhaustion

heat lamp
heating pad
heat prostration
heatstroke
hebephrenia
he'd**
hedonism
heed**
heel**
heel bone
Heimlich maneuver
heinous**
helico-**
helicoprotein
helio-**
heliotropic
helium
helix
he'll**
helminth-
helmintho-
helminthology
helper T cell
hema-
hemangioma
hemat/o-
hematein**
hematic
hematin**
hematinics
hematocrit test
hematology
hematoma**
hematophagous**
hematophagus**
hemi-
-hemia
hemicardia
hemihyperesthesia**
hemihypesthesia**
hemiplegia
hemisphere
hemizygous
hemo-
hemodialysis
hemogeneous**
hemoglobin
hemolysis

hemometer**
hemometra**
hemophilia**
hemophiliac**
hemophilic**
hemophilus
hemophobia**
hemoptysis
hemorrhage
hemorrhoids
hemostasis
hemostat
hemotherapy
hemp
henbane
Hensen**
heparin
hepat/o-
hepatectomy
hepatic
hepatitis
hepatitis B
hept/o-
herbal remedies
here**
hereditary
hereditary defect
heredity
hermaphrodite
hernia
herniated disk
heroin
herpes
herpes genitalis
herpes simplex
herpes zoster
hetero-
heterologous**
heteronomous**
heteronymous**
heterotopia**
heterotrophia**
heterotropia**
heterovaccine therapy
hexachlorophene
hexose sugar
hiatus
hiccup

hidr-
hidro-
high blood pressure
high-density lipoprotein
high-grade**
high grade**
high-tech product
hinge joint
hipbone
hip joint
Hippocratic oath
hirsutism
hist-
histamine
histidine
histo-
histocompatability antigens
histology
histoma**
histomine H
histone**
histoplasmosis
history
histotone**
histrionic personality
HIV antibody seronegativity
HIV antibody seropositivity
HIV asymptomaticity
HIV disease
hives
HMO
hoarse
Hodgkin's disease**
Hodgson's disease**
Hoechst-Roussel
Hoffman-La Roche
hol-
hole**
holism
holistic approach
holistic healing
holistic health
holistic medicine
hollow
holo-
holocrine
holocrine gland

holocrine secretion
holoenzyme
hom-
home/o-
homeopath
homeopathy
homeostasis
homicide
homo-
homocysteine**
homocystine**
homoerotic
homogeneous**
homol/o-
homologous**
homophobia**
homosexual
homozygote
honeymoon cystitis
hookworm
horizontal
hormonal therapy
hormone
hormone replacement therapy
Horneyhost surrogate
horny layer
horripilation
hospice
hospital
hospital administrator
hospital bed
hospitalization
hot flashes
hour**
house call
housemaid's knee
hue
human**
human chorionic gonadotropin
humane**
human immunodeficiency virus
humanistic psychology
human T-cell lymphocyte virus
humer-
humeral**
humero-
humerus**

humid
humor
humoral**
humoral immunity
humpback
humulene**
humulin**
humulus**
hunch**
hunchback
Huntington's chorea
hy-
hyal-
hyalo-
hydatid mole
hydr-
hydrastine**
hydrastinine**
hydrate
hydro-
hydrocele
hydrocephalus
hydrochloric acid
hydrogen peroxide
hydrolysis
hydrophobia
hydrostatic pressure
hydrotherapy
hydroxycorticosterone
hydroxydehydrocorticosterone
hydroxydesoxycorticosterone
hygiene
hymen
hyo-
hyoid
hyoscyamine
hyoscyamus
hyp-
hyper-
hyperacidity
hyperactive child syndrome
hyperbaric chamber
hyperbaric oxygenation therapy
hyperbaric therapy
hypercholesterolemia**
hypercholesterolia**
hyperchondrium

hyperemia
hyperglycemia**
hyperglycinemia**
hyperinsulinism
hyperlipidemia
hypermotility
hypernephroma
hyperopia
hyperphagia
hyperplasia
hyperpolarization
hypersensitivity
hypertension**
hyperthermia**
hypertonic solution
hypertrophy
hyperventilation
hypn/o-
hypnosis
hypnotic
hypnotics
hypo-
hypochlorous acid
hypocholesteremia
hypochondria
hypochondrium
hypodermic
hypodermic needle
hypodermic syringe
hypoglossal
hypoglossal nerve
hypoglycemia**
hypomanic personality
hypomotility
hypoplasia
hypopraxia
hypospadias
hypotension**
hypothalam/o-
hypothalamic-
hypothalamus
hypothermia**
hypothyroidism
hypotonic solution
hypoxia
hypoxic hypoxia
hyps/o-

hyster/o-
hysterectomy
hysteria

hysterical personality
hysterotrachelectomy**
hysterotrachelotomy**

I

-ia
-iac
I and D
-iasis
-iatric
iatro-
iatrogenic
-iatry
ibuprofen
-ic
ice pack
ichthulin
ichthy/o-
ichthyosis
-ics
icter/o-
ICU
id**
-id
I'd**
-ida
-idan
-idea
ideo-
ideopathic
idio-
idiocy
idiot
-idrosis
il-
ile/o-
ileac**
ileitis
ileostomy
ileum
ili/o-
iliac**
ilium
illness

illusion**
illusive**
im-
imbalance**
imipramine
immaturity reaction
immerse
immune responses
immune therapy
immunity
immunization
immunization therapy
immuno-
immunochemistry
immunoglobulin
immunology
immunomodulators
immunosuppressant
immunosuppressives
immunotherapy
impairment
impetigo
implant
implantation
impotence
impregnation
impulse
in-
inactive
in balance**
inborn error of metabolism
inborn immunity
incapacity
incest
incidence
incidents
incipient
incision
incision and drainage

incisor**
incisura**
incisure**
incoherence
incompatible
incompetent
incomplete
incontinence
incross**
incrust**
incubation period
incubator
incurable
incus
independent practice association
index finger
Indian hemp
indication
indigestion
indisposed
individual psychology
induced abortion
induration
industrial psychology
inebriated
inert
in extremis
infant
infantile paralysis
infantilism
infarction**
infect
infection
infectious
infectious disease
infer-**
inferior
inferiority complex
infertility
infestation
infiltrative
infirm
infirmary
infirmity
inflamed
inflammation
inflate
influenza

infra-**
infraction**
infrared therapy
infusion pump
ingredient
ingrown toenail
inhalant
inhalation
inhalator
inhale
inhaler
initial
inject
injection
injury
inner ear
innervate**
innocuous
innominate artery
innovate**
ino-
inoculation
inotropic agent
inpatient
inquest
insanity
insect
insecticide
insemination
inserts
inset
insist
in situ
insomnia
inspiration
inspirator
inspiratory reserve volume
instability
instep
instinct
instrument
insufficient
insulin
insulinase
insult
integumentary system
intensive care unit
inter-

inter-abdominal abscesses
intercellular fluid
intercostal muscle
intercostal nerve
intercourse
interface**
interferon
interior
interjection
intermediary
intermedin
intermission**
intermittent
intern**
internal cuneiform
internal environment
internal medicine
interne**
interneuron
internist
internuncial neuron
interphase**
interpose
interstitial cells
interstitial fluid
intertrigo
intervenous**
intervention
interventricular
intestin/o-
intestinal gas
intestinal juice
intestinal mucose
intestinal obstruction
intestine
intolerance
intoxicant
intra-
intramuscular
intrascleral
intrauterine device
intravenous**
intravenous infusion
intravenous therapy
intraventricular
intrinsic clotting pathway
intrinsic factor
intro-

introjection
intromission**
introversion
introvert
intubation
in turn**
in utero
invalid
invertase
invertebrate
in vitro
in vitro fertilization
involuntary muscle
involutional psychosis
iodide
iodine
iodoform
iodophors
iodotherapy
ionizing
ipecac
ipecacuanha
ir-
irid/o-
iridectomy
iridotomy
iris
iritis
iron
iron lung
irradiation
irregularity
irremeable**
irremediable**
irreversible
irrigate
irritability
irritable bowel syndrome
is/o-
ischemia
ischi/o-
ischium
ischomenia
Ishihara test
islets of Langerhans
-ism
isochromosome
isolation

isolation chamber
isolation ward
isoleucine
isometric contraction
isometric exercise
isoniazid
isopropyl
isotonic contraction
isotonic exercise
isotonic solution
-ist
isthmus of the uterine cavity

itching
-ite
-itic
-itis
IUD
iulio-
-ium
IV
IV needle
-ive
ivy pole

J

Jakob-Creutzfeldt
jalap
Jansen**
jaundice
jejun/o-
jejunum
jellies
Jensen**

jet lag
jimsonweed
Johnson & Johnson
joint disease
Jones
jugular trunk
Jung
Jungian psychology

K

Kahn
kala-azar
kanamycin
Kaposi's sarcoma
kary/o-
karyotype
Kegel exercises
kerat/o-
keratin
keratitis
keratolytics
keratoma
keratoplasty
keratosis**
keto-
ketone
ketosis**

kidney
kidney basin
kidney stone
killed-virus vaccine
kin/e/o-
kinesi/o-
kinesiology
kinesis
kinesthesia
kinetic
kinin
kissing disease
knee
knee brace
knock-knee
Knoll
knuckle

kola
kola nut
koro
Kotex
Krebs cycle
KUB

kwashiorkor
Kwell
KY jelly
kymograph
kyphosis

L

labia
labial**
labia majora
labia minora
labile**
labium
labor
laboratory technician
labored breathing
labyrinth
laceration
lacrim/o-
lacrimal**
lacrimale**
lacrimal gland
lact/i/o-
lactalbumin
lactase
lactation
lacteal gland
lactic acid
lactiferous sinus
lactigenic hormone
lactose
lacuna**
lacunar**
Laidlaw
Laidlow
La Leche League
-lalia
Lamaze
lameness
lamina**
laminar**
lance
lanced**

lancet**
Lange**
Langer**
Langerhans**
Langhans**
languishing
languor**
lanolin
laparo-
laparoscopy
laparotomy
laparotomy pack
lap pack
large intestine
laryng/o-
laryngectomy
laryngitis
laryngoscope
larynx
laser**
laser surgery
laser therapy
Lassa fever
lassitude
latency
latency leukoplakia
latent period
later/o-
lateral inhibition
latissimus dorsi
laudanum
laughing gas
lavage
laxative
lazar**
L-dopa

leach**
lead poisoning
leakage
learning disabilities
Leboyer
leche**
lecithin
lecithinase
lecithoprotein
Lederle
leech**
left-handed
leg
legionnaires' disease
leio-
lemon
lens
lentigo
leper**
lepo-
lepra**
leprosy
-lepsia
-lepsis
-lepsy
leptandra
lepto-
leptospira
leptospirosis
lesbian
lesion
lesser curvature
lethal dose
leuc/o-
leucine**
leucocyt-
leuk/o-
leukemia
leukin**
leukocyte
leukocyto-
leukocytosis
leukopenia
leukorrhea
lev/o-
level
levorphanol

levulose
-lexia
libido
Librium
licensed practical nurse
lid
lidocaine
lie**
life-support system
life-threatening
lifetime maximum
ligament**
ligamenta**
ligand
ligature
lightheadedness
limb
limbic system
limbus
linea**
lineae**
linear**
linen**
ling/i-
lingo-
lingual**
lingual braces
lingual papilae
lingula**
liniment
linin**
linkage
linoleic**
linolenic**
linolic**
lio-
lip/o-
lipa**
lipase
lipid
lipocaic
lipoma
lipoprotein
liposuction
lipoxidase
lippa**
lips**

liquid
liquid incense
lisps**
liter**
-lith
lithium
lithium carbonate
lithotomy
lithotripsy
lithotrite
litter**
little finger
liver**
liver spot
live virus vaccine
lividity
living will
livor**
lob/i/o-
lobe
lobes**
lobotomy
lobule**
lobuli**
lobus**
local**
local anesthetic
lochia
lochial**
lockjaw
locomotion
locus
log/o-
-logist
-logy
loin
loop**
loose**
lordosis
Lou Gehrig's disease
loupe**
louse
low blood pressure
low-density lipoprotein
lower extremities
low-grade fever
lozenge

LPN
LSD
lubricant
lues**
lumb-
lumbago
lumbar nerve
lumbar nodes
lumbar puncture
lumbar vertebrae
lumbo-
lumen
luminal**
Luminal**
lumpectomy
lung
lung cancer
lung surfactant
lupus
lupus erythematosus
lupus vulgaris
lute-
luteal phase
luteinizing hormone
luteo-
lycine**
lye**
Lyme disease
lymph
lymph-
lymphadenopathy syndrome
lymphatic drainage
lymphatic duct
lymphatic system
lymph gland
lymph node
lympho-
lymphocyte
lymphoid tissue
lymphokine
lymphoma
lyosol**
lys-
lysergic acid diethylamide
lysin**
-lysin
lysine**

-lysis
lyso-
Lysol**
lysosome

lysozyme
-lyte
-lytic
lyxose

M

Maalox
maceration
machine
macr-
macro-
macrobiotic
macrocephalous**
macrocephalus**
macrodactylia**
macrodactyly**
macrophage
macroprosopia
macroprosopy
macroscopic
macula**
macular**
macule**
mad itch
madman
Maganstrasse
maggot therapy
magnesia
magnesium
magnesium citrate
magnesium hydroxide
magnesium oxide
magnetic
magnetic resonance imaging
maieutic
maiming
mainstreaming
maintenance
major calyx
major medical
major surgery
mal**
mal-
malabsorption

malabsorption syndromes
malac-
-malacia
malaco-
maladie**
maladjustment
malady**
malaise
malar
malaria**
malariatherapy
male
male climacteric
male hypgonadism
male menopause
malformation
malfunction
malignancy
malignant
malignant coital headaches
malingering
Mall**
malleable
mallet
mallet finger
malleus
malnutrition
malocclusion
malpractice
malpractice insurance
maltase**
maltose**
malt sugar
mamm-
mamma
mamma-
mammary gland
mammi-

mammo-
mammogram
mammography
mammoplasty
mammotropic hormone
man**
managed care
mandible
mandibular
mandibular nerve
mandrel**
mandril**
mandrill**
mange
mania
-mania
manic depression
manic-depressive psychosis
manipulation
Mann**
manoever
manometer
manose
mantle
manual
manubrium
maple sugar
margin
marginal
margo
marijuana
marrow
marrow cavity
martyrdom
masculine
maser
masking of symptoms
mask of pregnancy
Maslow
masochism
mass
massage**
masseter
massive
massive bleeding
mast/o-
mast cell
mast cell stabilizers

mastectomy
master two-step test
-mastia
mastitis
mastoid
mastoidectomy
mastoid process
mastoplasia**
mastoplastia**
mastostomy**
mastotomy**
masturbation
mater
materia**
material**
materia medica
maternal
maternity
maternity hospital
matrix
mattress
maturation
mature
maturity
maxilla
maxillary nerve
maximal
maximum
MD
Mead-Johnson
meal
mean
measle**
measles**
measly**
measure
meatus
mechanical heart
mechanism
mechanoreceptor
mechanotherapy
meconium
medi-
media
medial
median
median cubital vein
median nerve

mediastinal
mediated transport
medic
Medicaid**
medical examiner
medical insurance
medically indigent
Medicare
medicate**
medicated dressing
medication
medicine
medio-
medium
MEDLARS
MEDLINE
medulla
medulla oblongata
medullary
megakaryocyte
megal-
megalo-
megalomaniac**
megalomanic**
megalopia**
megalopsia**
-megaly
meiosis**
melan-
melancholia**
melancholiac**
melancholic**
melanin
melano-
melanocyte
melanoma
melasma
melatonin
melibiose
Melissa
membrana**
membrane**
membranous
memory cell
men-
menacme
menarche
Mendel

mendelian laws
Ménière's syndrome
mening-
meningeal
meninges
meningi-
meningioma
meningitis
meningo-
meningococcal
meninx
menisous
meno-
menopausal
menopause
menorrhagia
menostatis
menoxenia
menses
menstrual cycle
menstrual extraction
menstrual flux
menstrual migraine
menstruation**
mensuration**
mental hospital
mental hygiene
mental illness
mentally
mental retardation
menthol**
Mentholatum
menthyl**
menticide
menton
mepazine
meperidine
meprobamate
merbromin
Merck
mercurial ointment
mercurials
mercuric chloride
Mercurochrome
mercurous chloride
mercury chloride
merocrine
merocrine gland

Merthiolate
mes/o-
mesatipellic
mesatipelvic
mescal
mescaline
mesenteric
mesh
mesio-
mesocolon
mesoderm
mesoglea**
mesoglia**
mesomorph
mesothelia**
mesothelial**
mesothelioma
mesovarian**
mesovarium**
message**
messenger RNA
met-
meta-
metabolic
metabolic acidosis
metabolic alkalosis
metabolic rate
metabolism
metacarp-
metacarpal
metacarpo-
metacarpus
metachromasia
metal
metamer**
metamere**
metamorphose**
metamorphosis**
metaphase
metaplasia
metaprotein
metapsychology
metastases**
metastasis**
metastasize
metatars-
metatarsal
metatarso-

metatarsus
*Metazoa***
metazoal**
-meter
methadone
methamphetamine hydrochlorate
methanal**
methanol**
Methedrine
methene**
methicillin
methine**
methionine
method
methodology
methyl
methylene blue
metopion**
metopium**
metopon**
metr-
metri-
metritis
metro-
metrodynia
metropexia
metropexy
metrorrhagia
-metry
Metycaine
micr/o-
microbe
microbicide
microbiology
microcephalic
microcephalous**
microcephalus**
microfilament
microfilaria
microglia**
microglial**
microorganism
microphage
microscope
microscopy
microsection
Microsporum
microsurgery

microsurgical free flap technique
microtome
microtubule
microwave diathermy machine
micturate
micturition
midbrain
middle cuneiform
middle ear
middle finger
midline
midtemporal
midwife
midwifery
migraine
migratory
mikvah
Miles
miliaria**
miliary**
milieu
milium
milk-free
milk leg
milk letdown reflex
milk of bismuth
milk of magnesia
milli-
milligram
Miltown
Minamata disease
mineral
mineralocorticoid
mineral oil
mineral water
miner's asthma
minimal brain dysfunction
minimum**
mini-pill
minium**
minor**
Minor**
minor calyx
minor operation
minor surgery
minor tranquilizer
miosis**
miotics

miracle drug
mirror imaging
miscarriage
misogamy**
misogyny**
missed
mitochondria
mitomycin
mitosis
mitral
mitral valve disease
mittelschmerz
mixture
MMR vaccine
mnemon
mnemonics
mobile
mobility**
Möbius
modal**
modality
mode
model**
moderate
modified radical mastectomy
moist wart
molar
molars
molasses
mold**
mole
molecular
molecule
molt**
mon-
monamine oxidase inhibitors
monaural
mongolism
*Monilia***
monilial**
monilial vaginitis
moniliasis
monitor
monkey virus
mono-
monoamine oxidase inhibitors
monochromat**
monochromate**

monococcus
monocular
monocyte
monogamy**
monogeny**
monogony**
monograph
monogyny**
monomania
mononuclear phagocyte system
mononucleosis
monophagia**
monophasia**
monosaccharide
monosynaptic reflex
monoxide
monozygotic
mons pubis
mons veneris
montage
monthlies
monthly period
mood
mood swings
morbid
morbidity
morbidity rate
morbific
morbus
morgue
moribund
morning-after pill
morning glory seeds
morning sickness
moron
morph-
-morph
morphea**
morphia**
-morphic
morphine
-morphism
morpho-
morphology
-morphy
mortality
mortify
mortuary

mosaic
mosquito
motility**
motion
motion sickness
motoneuron
motor
motor end plate
motor function
motor neuron
motor neuron diseases
mottling
moulage
mouth
mouthwash
movement
mRNA
muc-
muci-
mucilage
mucin
muco-
mucoid
mucopolysaccharide
mucopurulent
mucosa
mucosal
mucous**
mucous membrane
mucous plaque
mucus**
mucus observation
mulberry cell
multi-
multiaxial joint
multifactorial inheritance
multifocal mural
multiple
multiple personality
multiple sclerosis
multiplex
mumps
Munchausen syndrome
murmur
muscle
muscle-contraction headaches
muscle fatigue
muscle relaxer

muscle spasm
muscle spindle
muscle tone
muscul-
muscular
muscular atrophies
muscular dystrophy
muscularis
muscular system
musculo-
musculoskeleton
musculus
mustard plaster
mutagen
mutant
mutation
mute
muteness
mutilation
my-
myalgia
myalgic encephalomyelitis
myasthenia
myasthenia gravis
myatonia**
myc-
mycet/o-
mycetoma
-mycette
-mycin
myco-
mycobacteria
mycobacterium

mycology
mycomycin
mycoplasms
mycosis
mycotic
mye-
myel-
-myelia
myelin
myelin sheath
myelitis
myelo-
myeloma
Mylan
myo-
myocardial infarction
myocarditis
myocardium
myofibrils
myogenic
myoglobin
myoma
myopia
myopic
myosin
myotactic**
myotatic**
myotonia**
myx-
myxedema
myxo-
myxoid cyst

N

nabothian
nac-
naco-
NAD
naevose**
nail
nail-biting
nail fold
naked
nan-

nano-
nanus
nape
napkin
naphtha
narc-
narcissism
narcissistic
narco-
narcolepsy

narcotherapy
narcotic
nares
naris
narrowing
nas-
nasal
nasal cavity
nasal discharge
nasal sinus
nascent
nasi-
nasi plica
naso-
nasogastric
nasolabial sebaceous plugs
nasolacrimal duct
nasopharyngeal
nasopharynx
nasotrachial
nat-
natal
nati-
national health
National Institutes of Health
native dextran
nativism
natural childbirth
natural immunity
nature
naturopathic doctor
naturopathy
naupathia
nausea**
nausea gravidarum
nauseant
nauseated
navel
navel string
navose**
nearsighted
nearsightedness
nebulizer
neck
neck brace
necr-
necro-
necrophilia

necrophily
necrosis
necrotic**
needle
negative
negative feedback
negative test result
negligible
Neisseria
nemat-
nemato-
Nematoda**
nematode**
Nembutal
neoanalytic psychology
neocortex
neomycin
neonatal
neonate
neonatology
neonatorum
neoplasm
neoplasms
neoplastic
Neoprontosil
nephr-
nephralgia
nephrectomy
-nephric
nephritis
nephro-
nephrolithiasis
nephrolithotomy
nephrology
nephron unit
nephros
nephrosclerosis
nephrosis
nephrotoxic
nerv-
nerve**
nerve growth factor
nervi**
nervo-
nervosa angina
nervous**
nervous breakdown
nervous system

nervus**
nestitherapy
nestotherapy
neur-
neural
neuralgia
neural tube defect
neurasthenia
neurilemma**
neurilemmal**
neurit
neurite
neuritis
neuro-
neurodermatitis
neurofibromatosis
neurogenic
neurohypophyseal
neurohypophysial
neurologist
neurology
neuron
neuronal
neuropathy
neurorrhaphy
neurosis
neurosurgery
neurosyphilid**
neurosyphilis**
neurotic**
neurotica**
neurotic depression
neurotic-depressive reaction
neurotic disorder
neurotomy
neurotransmitter
neutral
neutralize
neutrophil
neutrophil exudation
nevose**
nevus**
newborn
niacin
niche
niche cell
nicotinamide adenine dinucleotide
nicotine

nictation
nictitation
night blindness
night-eating syndrome
nightmare
night sweats
night vision
nikethamide
nipa sugar
nipple
nit
nitrate**
nitride**
nitrite**
nitrogen
nitroglycerin
nitrous oxide
noble gas
noci-
nociceptor
noctambulism
nocturnal
nodal
node**
nodes of Ranvier
nodi**
nodosa
nodose**
nodosum
nodular
nodule
nodus**
-noia
noise
noma**
nomo-
-nomy
non-
nona**
nonaddicting
non compos mentis
noncontributory
nonfunctioning
noninfective state
noninvasive surgery
nonirritating diet
nonoperable tumor
nonpalpable

nonspecific
nonspecific surgery
nonspecific vaginitis
nonsterile
norepinephrine
norethynodrel
norgestrel
Norlestrin
norm-
normal
normally
normo-
normoactive
normoblast
northindrome
nos-
nose
nosebleed
noso-
nosocomial
nosology
nostril
not-
notch
not-for-profit
notifiable disease
notify
noto-
novobiocin
Novocain
noxious
NSAIDs
nucal
nucha
nuchal cord

nucle-
nuclear
nuclear envelope
nuclear medicine
nuclease
nuclei
nucleo-
nucleohistone
nucleolus
nucleoprotein
nucleotidase
nucleus
nulli-
nulligravida
nullipara
numb
numbness
nummular
Nupercaine
nurse
nurse-midwife
nurse-practitioner
nursery
nurse's aide
nursing home
nutrient
nutrition
nux vomica
nylon
nymph
nympho-
nymphomania
nystagmus
nystatin

O

o-
OB
obese
obesity
OB GYN
objective signs
oblique
obliquus

obliterans
obliteration
obsession
obsessive-compulsive neurosis
obsessive-compulsive
    psychoneurosis
obsessive-compulsive reaction
obsessive personality

obsolete
obstetrical
obstetrics
obstipation
obstruction
obturator
obtuse
occipital
occipital lobe
occiput
occlusal
occlusion
occlusive
occult blood
occupational therapy
occurring sporadically
octan**
octane**
ocular
oculi
oculo-
oculocardiac reflex
oculomotor nerve
od**
odd**
odont-
-odont
-odontia
odontitis
odonto-
odontoma
odor
odorous
-odynia
oedipal
Oedipus complex
oestrus**
*Oestrus***
office
-oid
oil gland
ointment
-ole
oleaginous
olfactory
olfactory lobe
olfactory nerve
olig-

oligo-
oligogenic**
oligogenics**
oligophrenia
olive oil
-oma
ombudsman
omega
omentum
omission**
omphal-
omphalo-
onanism
on-call
onch-
-onchia
oncho-
oncology**
onset
ontogeny
ontology**
onych-
-onychia
-onychium
onycho-
onychosis
onyxis
oo-
oocyte
oogamy
oogenesis
oophor-
oophorectomy
oophoro-
oosperm
opacification
opacity
opaque
open-heart surgery
operable cancer
operant
operating room
operation
operative
operative risk
ophthalm-
ophthalmia
-ophthalmia

ophthalmic nerve
ophthalmo-
ophthalmologist
ophthalmology
ophthalmoplegia
ophthalmoscope
-opia
opiate
opisth-
opistho-
opium
opponent
opportunist
opposing margins
-opsia
opsonic therapy
opsonins
opt-
optic
optic-
optical
optic chiasma
optician
optic nerve
optico-
optimal length
opto-
optometrist
optometry
or-
ora**
oral**
oral cavity
oral contraceptive
orale**
oral polio vaccine
oral surgeon
oral surgery
oral thermometer
orbicular
orbicularis
orbit
orbital**
orbital cavity
orbitale**
orchi-
orchid/o-
-orchidism

orchidotomy**
orchiectomy**
orchio-
orchiotomy**
-orchism
orchitis
orchotomy**
orderly
-orexia
organ
organ/o-
organelles
organic
organically
organic brain syndrome
organic disorder
organism
organ of Corti
organotherapy
organ system
organ transplant
orgasm
orgastic dysfunction
oriental
orifice
origin
original
oris
oro-
oropharyngeal
orphan
orrho-
orth-
ortho-
orthodiagraph
orthodontics
orthodontist
orthopedics
orthopedic surgeon
orthopnea
orthoptic**
orthoscope
orthostatic
orthotic**
orthotopic**
orthotropic**
oryzenin
os

oscillograph
-ose
-oses
-osis
-osises
osm-
-osmia
osmics
osmo-
osmolarity
osmoreceptor
osmosis
osmotic
osmotic pressure
osmotic shock
osse-
osseo-
osseomucoid
osseous
ossicular chain
ossificans
ossification
oste-
ostectomy
osteitis
osteo-
osteoarthritis
osteoblast
osteochondr-
osteochondro-
osteoclasis
osteoclast
osteologia**
osteology**
-osteoma
osteomyelitis
-osteon
osteopath
osteopathy
osteoporosis
osteotomy
ostia**
ostial**
ot-
otalgia
otherly abled
otic
-otic

otitis
oto-
otolaryngology
otology
otomycosis
otorhinolaryngology
otorrhea
otosclerosis
otoscope
ounce
our**
-ous
outbreak
outcropping
outer ear
outflow tract
outpatient
output
ova**
oval**
ovalbumin
oval window
ovar-
ovarian
ovarian follicle
ovaries
ovaro-
ovary
over**
overactive
overbite
overburdened heart
overcompensation
overdose
overflow
overlay
overprescribe
oversedation
overt
overweight
ovi-
oviduct
ovio-
ovocyte
ovoglobulin
ovoid**
ovotestis
ovovitellin

ovum
ox-
oxacillin
oxazepam
oxidative
oxidative fast fibers
oxidative phosphorylation
oxidative slow fibers
oxide
oxo-
oxygen

oxygenator
oxygen mask
oxygen tank
oxygen tent
oxygen therapy
oxyhemoglobin
oxyntic cells
oxytetracycline
oxytocic
oxytocin
ozone

P

pacemaker
pacinian corpuscle
pack
packed
Paddock
Paget's disease
-pague
pain
painful
painkiller
painless
pairs
palate
palatine
palatine tonsil
palato-
pale-
paleo-
palliative
palliative treatment
pallium
pallor
palmar
palm sugar
palpable
palpate**
palpation**
palpatory percussion
palpebral
palpila
palpitate**
palpitation**

palsy
pan-
panacea
pancreas
pancreat-
pancreatic amylase
pancreatic juice
pancreatitis
pancreato-
pancreozymin
pandemic**
P and V
panel
panic
pannus**
pant
pantaphobia**
pantophobia**
panus**
papain
Papanicolaou test
papaverine
papill/o-
papilla**
papillary
papilloma virus
papiniform plexus
pappose**
pappus**
Pap smear
Pap test
papula**

papular**
papule**
papulosa
par-
para
-para
para-
paracasein
parachymal
paracyesis**
paracytic**
paradox
paradoxical sleep
paraffin
paraglossa**
paraglossia**
parahormone
parakeratosis
paraldehyde
parallax
parallel
paralysis
paralytic
paramedic
parameter**
paranasal
paranoia
paranoid personality
paranoid schizophrenia
paraparesis
paraphilia
paraplegia
paraplexia
parapsychology
parasite**
parasitic**
parasitology
parasympathetic
parathyrin
parathyroid
parathyroid gland
parathyroid hormone
paratyphoid fever
paregoric
parenchyma
parenchymatous
parent
parenteral

paresis**
parietal
parietal cells
parietal lobe
Parke-Davis
parkinsonism
Parkinson's disease
paro-
parotid
parotid gland
-parous
paroxysm
paroxysmal
pars
partes**
parthenogenesis
partial
partially
partition
parts**
parturition
passage
passed**
passive-aggressive personality
passive-aggressive reaction
passive-dependence reaction
passive immunity
passive smoking
past**
paste**
Pasteurella
patch
patch test
patell/o-
patella**
patellar**
patency
patent**
patent medicine
paternity
path-
-path
-pathia
-pathic
patho-
pathogen
pathogenic
pathogens

pathologic
pathologist
pathology
pathomimicry
pathway
-pathy
patient**
patient advocacy
patten**
pattern**
paunch**
Pavlov
peak**
pear-shaped heart
pecten**
pectin**
pectoral
pectoral fascia
pectoral girdle
pectoris
pectous**
pectus**
ped-
pedal
pediatric
pediatrics
pedicule
pediculosis
pediculosis pubic
pediculous**
pediculus**
pedio-
pedo-
pedodontics
pedophilia
peduncule
peek**
peeling of skin
peer review organization
peg
pelada
pelade
pellagra
-pellic
pellicula**
pellicular**
pelv-
pelves**

pelvi-
pelvic
pelvic girdle
pelvic inflammatory disease
pelvis**
pemphigus
pen-
pendulous
penetrance
-penia
penicillin
penile
penile prosthesis
penis
peno-
pentobarbital
pentosan
pentose sugar
Pentothal
-pepsia
pepsin
peptic ulcer
peptidase
peptide
Pepto-Bismol
peptone
peptones
per**
per-
perception
percussion
percussion hammer
percutaneous
perennial
perforated
perforation
perfusion**
Pergonal
peri-
perianal
periaortic
pericardial cavity
pericardial disease
pericarditis
pericardium
pericyte**
perimeter**
perinatal**

perinatology
perineal**
perineum
period
periodic
periodontal disease
periodontal membrane
periodontics
periodontist
periosteal
periosteum
peripheral
peripheral resistance
peristalsis
peristaltic waves
periton-
peritonitis
peritono-
peritoneal**
permanent
permeable
permissiveness
pernicious anemia
peroneal**
peroneal nerve
peroxide
peroxisome
perphenazine
persecution complex
persistent
personal**
personal health care
personal indifference
personality disorder
personality theory
personnel**
person with AIDS
perspiration
pertussis
pervert
pervious**
pes**
pessary
pest**
pesticide
pestilence
petit mal
petrolatum

petroleum jelly
petrosa**
petrosal**
PET scan
-pexy
peyote
Pfizer
phac-
phaco-
phag-
phage
-phagia
-phagic
phago-
phagocyte
phagocytosis
-phagy
phak-
phako-
phalang-
phalangeal**
phalanges
phalango-
phalanx
phallic symbol
phallo-
phanazone
phantom limb
pharmac/o-
pharmaceutical
pharmacist
pharmacologist
pharmacology
pharmacopoeia
pharmacotherapy
pharmacy
pharyng-
pharyngeal**
pharyngitis
pharyngo-
pharyngopalatine arch
pharynx
phase
-phasia
phasic
phaso-
phenacetin
phencyclidine

phenelzine
phenethicillin
phenobarbital
phenocopy
phenoglycodal
phenol
phenolphthalein
phenols
phenomenological approach
phenomenon
phenothiazine
phenotype
phenyl**
phenylalanine
phenylketonuria
phenyl salicylate
pheochromocytoma
pheromone
phial**
-phil
-phile
-philiac
philtrum
phimosis
phleb/o-
phlebitis
phlebogram
phlebotomy
phlegm**
phlegmatic
phlegmonous
phloem**
-phobe
phobia
-phobia
phobic
-phobic
phobic reaction
phonation**
phonetic
phonocardiogram
phonocardiography
phonogram
-phony
-phoria
phosphate
phosphene**
phosphine**

phosphoaminolipide
phosphoglucomutase
phospholipid
phosphoprotein
phosphorus
phosphorylase
phosphorylation
photic
photo-
photogen**
photogene**
photopic vision
photopigment
photoplethysmograph
photoreceptor
phototherapy
phrase**
phren-
phrenia-
phrenic
phreno-
phthalylsulfathiazole
phthisis
phylogeny
phylum**
physi-
physiatrics**
physiatrist**
physic**
physical**
physically
physical medicine
physical therapist
physical therapy
physician
physician liability
physio-
physiologic
physiological
physiology
physiopathology
physiotherapist
physiotherapy
physique**
phyt-
phyto-
pia**
pial**

pica
picrotoxin
pigeon toes
pigment
pigmentation
pigmentory
pigmentosa
pil-
piles
pili-
piliated
pill
pillar
pilo-
piloerection
pilomotor
pilonidal
pilose**
pilus**
pimple
pineal body
ping-pong infection
pink disease
pinkeye
pinna
piperocaine
pique**
piriform
pisiform
piston
Pitocin
pitressin
pituitary
pituitary gland
pityriasis
pivot joint
placebo
placement
placenta
placentae bruit
placentation
plague
plain gut
plane
plane wart
Planned Parenthood Federation
planning
planta**

plantar**
plantar flexors
plantar wart
plaque
-plasm**
plasma**
plasma cell
plasma extender
plasma fractions
plasma membrane
plasma transfusion
plasmid
plasmin
Plasmodium malariae
plaster
plastic surgery
plastid
plate
platelet
platyopic
-plegia
plessor
pleur-
pleura
pleural**
pleural cavity
pleurisy
pleuritic**
pleuro-
plexor
plexus
plexuses
plica
plumbism
plural**
pneum/o-
pneumatic
pneumatograph
pneumatometer
pneumococcal infections
pneumococcus microorganism
pneumoconiosis
Pneumocystis carinii pneumonia
pneumogastric nerve
pneumogram
pneumograph
pneumonectomy
pneumonia

pneumoniae
pneumonic plague
pneumonitis
pneumothorax
pnigphobia
pock
pocked**
pocket**
pockmark
pocks**
podagra
podiatry
podophyllin
point
poison**
poisoning
poison ivy
poisonous
poison sumac
Poisson**
polar
polarizing
poles**
polio
poliomyelitis
polio vaccine
polishing
Pollack
Pollak
pollution
polus**
poly-
polychromatic
polycystic
polydipsia
polyethylene
polymorph
polymorphonuclear granulocytes
polymorphous perverse
polymyxin
polyneuritis
polynucleotidase
polyp
polypectomy
polypeptide
polypoid
polypous**

polypus**
polysaccharidea
polyunsaturated fat
polyuria
pons
pontine
popliteal
popliteal nerve
poppers
pore**
porous**
porphyria
portal system
porus**
positive
positive bone scan
positive feedback
positive test result
positron emission tomograph
possible diagnosis
post-
posterior
posterior chamber
posterior lobe disorders
posthumous
postmortem
postnasal drip
post-op
postoperative
postpartum
postpartum depression
postprandial
postsurgical
postsynaptic neuron
post-term birth
posttraumatic
posttraumatic stress syndrome
postural back problem
posture sense
potassium
potassium permanganate
potent
potential
potentiation
poultice
pouch
pour**

pox**
practical nurse
practice
practitioner
praecox
pre-
pre-AIDS
precancerous
precardial vein
precaution
precocious puberty
precordial
predisposing cause
predisposition
prednisone
predominant
preeclampsia
preexisting condition
preferred provider organization
pregnancy test
pregnant
preliminary
premature
premature birth
prematurely
premenstrual syndrome
premolar
prenatal**
preoperative
prep
preparation
prepped
prepuce
presacral
presbyopia
prescribed
prescription
presenile
presenile dementia
presentation
pressor**
pressure**
pressure point technique
presumptive
presynaptic neuron
presystolic murmur
preterm

prevalence
prevention
preventive
preventive medicine
previous**
priapism
prickly heat
primary
primary care
primary care network
primitive
principal**
principle**
prion
prior
prism
private duty nurse
private hospital
private insurance
private practice
pro-
proband
probe
probing of wound
problem
procaine
procedure
procedure capture
process
processes
processus
prochlorperazine
procrastination
proct-
proctalgia fugax
procto-
proctology
proctoscope
product line extension
professional career
profuse
profusion**
progesterone
progestin
prognosis
programmed
progression

215

progressive
prohormone
projection
prokaryote
prolactin
prolamin
prolapse
proliferation
proline
prolonged labor
promazine
prominent anthelix
pronation**
prone
Prontosil
pronucleus
propane**
propene**
prophase
prophylactic
prophylaxis
proprioception
proptosis
prospective payment
prostaglandin
prostate**
prostate gland
prostatic cancer
prostatitis
prosthesis
prosthodontics
prosthodontist
prostrate**
prostration
prot-
protamine
protean**
protease
protein**
proteinase
protein supplement
protein therapy
proteolipid
proteolipide
proteolytic
proteose**
proteus**

prothrombin
protime
proto-
protocol
protoplasm
protoxide of nitrogen
*Protozoa***
protozoal**
protozoal diseases
protrusion
protuberance
provider
proximal
prune juice sputum
pruritic**
pruritic rash
pruritus
pruritus ani
Prussack**
prussic**
-pselaphesia
pseud-
pseudo-
pseudomallei
pseudomembranous
Pseudomonas
pseudomucinous
pseudoparalysis
pseudopregnancy
pseudotabes
pseudotuberculosis
psi
psilocin
psilocybin
psilosis
psoas
psora
psoriasis
psych-
psychasthenia
psyche
psychedelic
psychiatric
psychiatry
psychic**
psycho-
psychoactive

psychoanalysis
psychoasthenic reaction
psychobabble
psychobiology
psychodelic
psychodrama
psychogenic
psychological dependency
psychology
psychomotor
psychoneurosis
psychoneurotic disorder
psychopathic personality
psychopathology
psychopharmacology
psychophysics
psychophysiological
psychophysiology
psychosensory disturbance
psychosexual disorder
psychosis**
psychosomatic
psychosomatic disorder
psychosomatic illness
psychosurgery
psychotherapeutic drugs
psychotherapist
psychotherapy
psychotic
psychotropics
psyllium**
psyllium seed
pterin**
pterion**
pterygium
-pterygium
pterygoid
ptoma-
ptomaine
ptosis
ptotic kidney
ptyalin
-ptyosis
-ptysis
puberty
pubes**
pubic lice

pubic symphysis
pubis**
public health
Public Health Nurse
Public Health Service
pubococcygeal muscle
pubococcygeus
pubovaginal muscle
pudendal block
puer-
puerperal fever
puerperal infection
puerperium
pull
pulm-
pulmo-
pulmonary
pulmonary artery
pulmonary embolism
pulmonary function test
pulmonary vein
pulmonary ventilation
pulmonic valve disease
pulmotor
pulp**
pulp canal
pulp chamber
pulpa**
pulpal**
pulsating
pulsation
pulse
pulse pressure
pulse rate
pulses
pulsus
pulvis**
punch**
punctate
punctum
puncture
pupal
pupil**
pupillae
pupillary
Purdue Frederick
pure**

217

purgative
purge
purine
purine bases
purpura
purr**
purulent
pus
pus basin
pustulant
pustular
pustule
putrescence
putrid bronchitis
P wave
py-
pyel-
pyelo-
pyelogram
pyelography
pyelonephritis
pyloric
pyloroplasty
pylorus

pyo-
pyocyanas
pyocyanase
pyocyanin
pyogenes**
pyogenic**
pyogens**
pyorrhea
pyosalpinx
pyr-
pyramid
pyramidal neuron
pyramidon
pyrectic**
pyretic**
pyrexia**
pyrexial**
pyriform
pyro-
pyrogenic**
pyroretotherapy
pyrosis
pyrrole
pyuria

Q

Q fever
QRS complex
Q-T interval
Quaalude
quack
quackery
quad-
quadrant
quadrate lobe
quadri-
quadriceps
quadrilateral
quadriplegia
quality
quantitative
quantity
quarantine
quart
quartan
quarter evil

quarternary ammonia compounds
quartz lamp
quassia
querulent
questionable
quickening
quiescent
quietly
quinacrine
Quincke**
quinidine
quinine
quinolones
quinque**
quinsy
quintuplet
quotidian ague
quotient
qv
Q wave

R

rabbit**
rabbit test
rabid**
rabies
race
rachi/o-
rachitic scoliosis
racket amputation
racquet incision
radi/o-
radia fossa
radial nerve
radian**
radiant**
radiant heat
radiating
radiation
radiation keratotomy
radiation sickness
radiation therapy
radical**
radical mastectomy
radical treatment
radicular pain
radiculopathy
radicle**
radioactive
radiobe**
radiode**
radiodontist
radiographer
radiography
radioisotope
radio knife
radiological
radiologist
radiolucent
radiopaque
radiopharmaceuticals
radiotherapist
radiotherapy
radium therapy
radius
radix
raffinase**
raffinose**

raise**
rale
rami
ramose**
ramus**
rapid eye movement
rash
rasion**
rasp
raspatory**
ratio
ration**
rationalization
rauwolfia
Rauwolfia derivative
Raynaud's disease
rays**
raze**
re**
re-**
Re
reaction formation
reactive disorder
reactive hyperemia
reactivity
Read method
reagent**
reagin**
real anxiety
reattachment
recent
reception
receptive
receptor
receptor potential
recess**
recession
recessive
recessive trait
recessus**
recipient
reciprocal
recombinant DNA
recombination
recommended dietary allowance
reconstruction

reconstructive surgery
record**
recovery room
recrudescence
recruitment
rect/o-
rectal thermometer
rectocele
rectostomy**
rectotomy**
rectovaginal examination
rectum
rectus abdominus
rectus femoris
recumbent
recuperation
recurrence
recurrent
red blood cell
red blood count
red currant jelly sputum
red muscle fibers
reduced hemoglobin
reduction
redundant
reefer**
refer**
reference
referral
referred pain
reflects**
reflex**
reflex arc
reflux**
refraction
refractory period
refractured
refusal
regime
regimen
regio**
region**
regional block
regiones
registered nurse
regression
regular rhythm

regurgitant esophagitis
regurgitation
rehabilitation
rehabilitation medicine
reimbursement
reinforcement
rejection
relapse
relapsing fever
relative
relative refractory period
relaxant
relaxation relief
relaxed pelvic floor
release
relevant**
relief**
relieve**
remedy
remission
remittant fever
removal
REM sleep
renal
renal calculus
renal colicretinitis pigmentosa
renal pelvis
reni-
renin**
renio-
rennin**
reparative
repetitive
replacement therapy
reportable disease
repositor**
repository**
repression
reproductive system
research
resection
resectoscope
resentment
reserpine
reservoir
resident
residual**

residual volume
residue**
resins
resistance
resistant
resonance
resorcinol
respiration
respirator
respiratory**
respiratory acidosis
respiratory alkalosis
respiratory arrest
respiratory distress syndrome
respiratory quotient
respirometer
response
rest home
resting membrane potential
restlessness
rest pain
restraint
restriction
result
resuscitation
resuscitator
retail customer
retained
retainer
retardation
retarded
rete
retention
rete testis
reticular
reticulose**
reticulosis**
reticulum
retin/o-
retina**
Retin-A**
retinal**
retinitis
retinopathy
retraction sign
retractor
retro-

retrocolic**
retrocollic**
retroflexed
retrograde
retroperitoneal
retrospective
retrospective billing
retrosternal
retroverted
retroverted uterus
retroviral
retrovirus
retrovirus inhibitor
revascularization
revellent**
reversed
reverse tolerance
reversion
revolution
Reye's**
Reye's syndrome
Rh**
rhabd/o-
rhamnose**
*Rhamnus***
-rhaphy
rhe**
rheo-
rhesus factor
rheum**
Rheum**
rheumatic fever
rheumatic heart disease
rheumatism
rheumatoid arthritis
rheumatology
Rh factor
rhin/o-
rhinitis
rhinolith
rhinoplasty
rhinorrhea
rhizotomy
rhod-
rhodo-
rhomboid
rhonchal

rhonchial
rhonchus
rhythmical tremor
rhythmic chorea
rhythm method
rhytidectomy
rib
rib beading
ribbon muscles
riboflavin
ribonuclease
ribonucleic acid
ribose
ribosome
Richardson Vicks
rickets**
*Rickettsia***
rickettsiae
rickettsial diseases
Ricord**
rictus
ridge
ridged**
right**
right atrium
right ventricle
rigid**
rigidity of muscles
rigor mortis
ring chromosome
ring finger
ringworm
risk
rite**
Robins
Roche
Rochelle powders
Rocky Mountain spotted fever
rod
roentgen
roentgeno-
roentgenography
roentgenoscope
Rolaids
rolfing
Rollet**

Rollett**
rongeur
room**
root**
root canal
root sheath
Rorschach
rosacea
rosein**
roselle**
roseola**
rosin**
Ross
rotary
rotation
rotator cuff
rotatory
rotavirus
roughage
rough endoplasmic reticulum
rounds
route**
routine
Roux**
-rrhage
-rrhagia
-rrhea
RU-486
rubber**
rubber gloves
rubefacient
rubella**
rubeola**
ruber**
rubin
Rubin
rubor**
rue**
rugae
rugal
running
runny nose
rupture
ruptured disc
rusty sputum

S

Sabin vaccine
sac**
saccharase
saccharide group
saccharifying enzyme
saccharin**
saccharine**
saccharose
sacculated aneurysm
saccule**
sacculi**
sacculus**
Sachs**
sack**
sacr/o-
sacral nerve
sacral vertebrae
sacrococcygeal
sacrogenital fold
sacroiliac
sacrum
sacs**
saddle block
sadism
sadomasochism
safe
sagittal sinus
Saint Vitus' Dance
sal ammoniac
salapingotomy
salicylic acid
saline
saline solution
saliva
salivary amylase
salivary glands
Salk vaccine
salmine
salmonella
Salmonella
salmonella poisoning
salol
salping-
salpingectomy

salpingitis
salpingo-
salpingo-oophorectomy
salpingopalatine fold
salts
salve**
*Salvia***
sample
sanative
sanatory**
sandfly fever
Sandoz
sanguin/o-
sanguineous
sanguinous
sanitary**
sanitary napkin
sanitorium
Sanofi Winthrop
sapr/o-
saprophyte
sarc-
sarcina
sarco-
sarcoid
sarcoma
sarcomere
sarcosine
sartorius
sassafras
satellite
satisfactorily
satisfactory
saturated fat
saturation
satyriasis
save**
saw**
scab
scabbing
scabetic infection
scabicides
scabies
scald

scale
scalene
scaler
scalp
scalpel
scan
scaphoid
scapul/o-
scapula**
scapular**
scar**
scare**
scarlatina
scarlet fever
scatoma**
Schering
-schisis
schist/o-
schistosomiasis
schizo-
schizoid
schizoid personality
schizokinesis
schizophrenia
schizophrenic patient
schizothymia
schizotypal personality
Schmutz pyorrhea
Schultz
Schultze
Schwann's cells
sciatica
sciatic nerve
scientific
scirrhous**
scirrhus**
scissors
scler/o-
sclera
sclerae
scleral
scleral crescent
sclerectoiridectomy
sclerectomy
scleroderma
sclerose**
sclerosed
sclerosis

-sclerosis
sclerous**
sclerous tissues
scrofula
scoliosis
scoop
scop/o-
-scope
-scopic
scopolamine
-scopy
score
scotoma**
scourge
scrape
scraping
scratch
scratch test
screen
screening
screw
scrofulous
scrot/o-
scrotal
scrotum
scrub nurse
scrub suit
scurf
scurvy
seagull murmur
seal
seamless
Searle
seasickness
seasonal affective disorder
sebaceous cyst
sebaceous gland
seborrhea
seborrheic dermatitis
sebum
secobarbital sodium
Seconal
secondary care
second-degree burn
secreta**
secrete**
secretin**
secretion**

secretory vesicles
section
sector iridectomy
sedation
sedative
sedimentation rate
SED rate
seed graft
seeing eye dog
segmental
segmentation
segmented
segmentum
segregation
Seidlitz powders
seizure
selective arteriography
self-infection
self-treatment
self-victimization
sella**
sellar**
seltzer
semeiology
semeiotics
semen**
semi-
semicircular canal
semilunar
semin/o-
seminal vesicle
seminiferous tubules
semiology
semiotics
semipermeable membrane
Semon**
senescence
senile
senile dementia
senile psychosis
senilis
senility
senna
sensation
sense organs
senses**
sensibility
sensitive

sensitivity
sensitization
sensor**
sensory receptors
sentinel polyp
separate pockets of pus
separating saw
separation
sepsis
septal deviation
septic
septic abortion
septicemia
septicemic meningitis
septum
sequence pyelogram
sequential oral contraceptives
ser-
serial**
series
serine
serious**
sero-
serologic
serological
serological tests
serology
seromuscular
seronegativity
seropositivity
seropurulent discharge
seroreaction
serosa
serosal
serotherapy
serotonin
serous**
Serpasil
serrated**
Sertoli's cell
serum**
serum albumin
serum cholesterol
serum globulin
serum hepatitis
serum transfusion
service
session

severance
severe
severed tendon
severity
sex change operation
sex chromatin
sex chromosome
sex-limited
sex-linkage
sex reassignment surgery
sexual dimorphism
sexually transmitted disease
shadow cell
shaft
shaking palsy
shallow breathing
shank
sharp pain
sheaf
sheath**
sheathe**
Shiatsu
shield
shift-shin splint
Shigella
shigellosis
shinbone
shingles
shivers
shock
shock reaction
shock therapy
shoddy**
shortening reaction
short pulse
shortwave diathermy machine
shot
shotty**
shoulder
shoulder blade
shunt
sial-
sialo-
Siamese twins
sib
sibling
sick bay
sick bed

sickle-cell
sickle-cell anemia
sickle scaler
sickness
sick room
SIDA
side effect
sider/o-
siderosis
siderotic nodules
SIDS
SIECUS
sight**
sigmoid colon
sigmoid flexure
sigmoidoscope
sign**
signal node
significance
significant pathway
silent carcinoma
silhouette
silic/o-
silicon**
silicone**
silicone-gel implant
silicone implant
silicosis
silk suture
silkworm gut
silver protein
simple fracture
simplex
simulate**
simultaneous
sine**
sine wave
single harelip
single photon emission computed
    tomography
singultus
sinoatrial node
sinoauricular
sinuous**
sinus**
sinusitis
sinusoidal
sinus rhythm

site**
sitology**
situation
situational psychosis
sitz bath
skeletal
skeleton
Skene's ducts
skenitis
skin
skin eruption
skin graft
Skinner
skipped beat
skull
slash
sleep and dreams
sleeping pill
sleeping sickness
sleepwalking
slice
sliding-filament mechanism
slightly
sling
slipped disc
slough
slow-wave sleep
sluggish reaction
slurred speech
small intestine
smallpox
smear
smegma
smelling salts
SmithKline Beecham
smooth endoplasmic reticulum
smooth muscles
snail fever
snare
sneeze
sniffle
snore
socialized medicine
social psychology
sociopath
socket
sodium
sodium amobarbital

sodium bicarbonate
sodium bromide
sodium hydroxide
sodium hypochlorite
sodium phosphate
sodium salicylate
soft palate
soft tissue
soft tissue damage
sol**
solar plexus
sole**
soleus
solitary nodule
soluble insulin
solution
soma**
soma-
somat/o-
somatic delusion
somatic receptor
somatization disorder
somatoform disorder
somatogenic psychosomatic
    disorder
somatoplasm
somatopsychology
somatotropin
somatotropic hormone
-somia
somnambulism
somni-
somnolent
son/o-
sonogram
soor**
soporific
sorbose
sore**
souffle
soul**
sound
space
space medicine
Spanish fly
spasm
-spasm
spasmodic

spastic colon
spastic contractures
spasticity
spatia**
spatial**
spatial summation
spatula
specialist
species
specific dynamic action
specificity
specific therapy
specimen
specimen bottle
spectinomycin
speculum
speech disorders
speech dysfunction
spell
sperm
sperm-
sperma-
spermat/o-
spermatic cord
spermatogenesis
spermatozoon
sperm count
spermi-
spermicidal jelly
spermicide
spermo-
sphenoid
sphenoidal
sphere
spherical aberration
spheroid joint
sphincter
sphygmograph
sphygmomanometer**
sphygmometer**
spica of the shoulder
spicula**
spicule**
spike pattern
spiking dysrhythmia
spilled protein
spina bifida
spinal accessory nerve

spinal column
spinal cord
spinal meningitis
spindle
spindle fibers
spine
spinnbarkeit
spiral
spirilla
spirillum
spirits of camphor
spiro-
spirochete
spirograph
spirometer
splanchnic
spleen
splen/o-
splenic
splicing
splint
split brain
split personality
splitting
spondyl/o-
spondylitis
spondylosis
sponge
spongy bone
spontaneous abortion
spor/i/o-
sporadic
spore
sports medicine
spotted fever
spotting
sprain
sprue
spur
sputum
squama**
squame**
squamous cell
squint
stabile**
stable**
stadium
staff**

stage
stain
staining
standard
standstill
stapes
staph**
Staphcillin
staphyl/o-
staphylococci
staphylococcus
starch
stasis
-stasis
stat**
-stat
state**
static
status
steady state
stearoyl**
steat/o-
stella**
stellar**
stellate
stem
stenosis
stent
sterile**
sterile saline solution
sterility
sterilization
stern/o-
sternal
sternoclavicular
sternocleidomastoid
sternotomy
sternum
sternutation
steroid
sterol**
stertorous respiration
stethograph
stethometer
stethoscope
stiffness
stilbestrol
stillborn

stimulant
stimulate**
stimulation
stimulus
stirrups
stitch
stitches
stoma**
stomach
stomachache
stomach pump
stomach tube
stomat/o-
stomatitis
-stomy/-stomies
stone
stool
stoop**
strabismus
straight
strain
straitjacket
stramonium
strangury
strategy
stratum corneum
stratum germinativum
stratum granulosum
stratum lucidum
strawberry mark
strength
strenuous exercise
strep throat
strepto-
streptococcal sore throat
streptococci
streptococcus
streptomycin
streptothricin
stress
stress fracture
stress incontinence
stress management
stress reaction
stress receptor
stress test
stretcher
stretch marks

229

stria
striae
striated muscle
stricture**
stridor
strip**
stripe**
stroke
stroke volume
stroma**
stromal
structuralism
structure**
struma**
strychnine
stub
stump
stunt
stupe**
stupor
stupp**
sturine
stutter
stuttering
sty
stye
stylet
styloglossus
stylohyoid
stylomastoid
sub-
subacute
subaortic
subarachnoid
subatomic
subcapsular
subclavian
subclavian trunk
subclavicular murmur
subclinical
subconscious
subcostal
subcutaneous
subcutaneous fat
subcuticular
subdermal
subdural
subdural hematoma

subjective
sublimation
sublime**
subline**
sublingual gland
subluxation
submandibular
submaxillary gland
submental
submitted
submucosal
submucous
subnormal
subnormality
substance
substance abuse disorder
substantia**
substantial**
substernal
substitution
substitution therapy
substrate
subtilin
succinylsulfathiazole
succus**
succus entericus
succuss**
sucrase**
sucrose**
suction
sudden
sudden infant death syndrome
sufficient
suffocation
sugar
suggestion therapy
suicidal
suicide
sulcus
sulfa**
sulfadiazine
sulfadimethoxine
sulfaguanidine
sulfa level
sulfamerazine
sulfanilamide
sulfapyrazine
sulfapyridine

Sulfasuxidine
Sulfathalidine
sulfathiazole
sulfisoxazole
sulfo-**
sulfonamide
sulfonethylmethane
sulfur**
Sullivan
Sullivanian theory
summa
summation
sunburn
sunstroke
super-
superficial
superficial infections
superior
superiority complex
supernumerary
supervision
supervisor
supine
supplement
support
supportive
suppository
suppression
suppressor T cell
suppurating gastritis
suppuration
supra-
supraclavicular
supraorbital
suprapatellar
suprapubic
suprarenal
suprarenal gland
suprascapular
supratrochlear
supraventricular
surface
surfactant
surfer's knot
Surgeon General
surgery
surgery consent form
surgical dressing

surgical gloves
surgical gown
surgical instruments
surgical mask
surgical needle
surgical sponge
surgical staple
surgicenter
surgicotherapy
surrogacy
surrogate
surrogate mother
surroundings
surveillance
survey
survival
susceptibility
susceptible
suspension
suspensory
suspicious
sustained cardiac arrest
sutura
suture
sutured
suture needle
swab
swallow
swallowing
swayback
sweat
sweat gland
sweating
swelling
swollen
sycosis**
Sydenham's chorea
sylvian
sym-
symbiosis
symmetrical
symmetry
sympathetic
sympatholytic
symphysis
symptom
symptomatic
symptomatology

syn-
synapse**
synapsis**
synaptic cleft
synchronous
syncope
syndesm/o-
syndrome
synergism
synergistic muscle
synergy
syngamy
synotosis
synovial
synovial capsule

Syntex
synthesis
synthetic
synthetic reactions
syntone
syphilis
syphilitic
syringe
syrup of ipecac
system
systematic
systemic
systemic circulation
systole
systolic pressure

T

tabasheer
tabes dorsalis
tabetic gait
table
tablet
tache**
taches**
tachy-
tachycardia
tachyphagia**
tachyphasia**
tachypnea
tactile
taen-
taeni-
taenia**
*Taenia***
tagatose
TAH-BSO
tail
tailbone
talipes
talo
talose**
talus**
tamarin**
tamarind**
tampan**

tampon**
tamponade
T and A
tantalum
tape
taper**
tapering
tapeworm
tapir**
tardive dyskinesia
tare**
target
tars/o-
tarsal
tarsus
tartar
taste bud
tattoo surgery
taxonomy
Tay-Sachs disease
TB
T cell
tea
teaching hospital
tear** (pron. *tare*)
tear** (pron. *teer*)
tear duct
tear gland

tears**
teat
technic**
technique**
teeth**
teethe**
Teflon implant
tegmental
tel/o/e-
tela**
telangiectasia
telephase
teller**
temperature
template
temple
tempora**
temporal**
temporal lobe
temporal summation
temporary
ten-
tenaculum
tend-
tendency
tenderness**
tendinitis**
tendinous**
tendo-
tendomucin
tendon
tendonitis**
tenesmus
tennis elbow
teno-
tenonitis**
tense
tenser**
tension headaches
tensor**
tensure**
tentative diagnosis
tentinous**
tepid
terapsin
terat-
terato-
teratogen

teratology
teratoma
tere**
teres**
term
terminal
terminal illness
terpene**
terpin**
Terramycin
tertiary care
tertiary syphilis
test-
testes**
testicle
testicul-
testiculo-
testis**
testo-
testosterone
testosterone deficiency syndrome
tests**
test-tube baby
tetanic**
tetanic convulsion
tetanus
tetanus toxin
tetany
tetra-
tetracaine
tetracycline
tetrahydrocannabinol
thalamic
thalamus
thalidomide
thalassemia
thanat-
thanato-
thanatos
theca
thelarche
thelitis
theoretical psychology
therapeutic abortion
therapeutics
therapeutic window
therapist
therapy

therm-
thermal
-thermia
-thermias
-thermies
thermo-
thermogenesis
thermometer
thermophilic**
thermophylic**
thermoreceptor
-thermy
thesis
theta
thiamin**
thiamine**
thickened
thickening
thick filaments
thigh
thighbone
thimerosal
thin filaments
thio-**
thiol**
thiopental sodium
thioridazine
thioxanthenes
third
third-degree burn
thirst
thorac-
thoraci-
thoracic
thoracic cavity
thoracic nerve
thoracic vertebrae
thoraco-
thoracoplasty
thoracostomy
thoracotomy
thorax
Thorazine
threatened labor
threonine
threshold
-thrix
throat

throbbing
throe**
thromb-
thrombin
thrombo-
thrombocyte
thrombocytosis
thromboembolism
thrombophlebitis
thrombosis
thrombus
throw**
throw up
thrush
thumb
-thymia
thymin**
thymine**
thymion**
thymol
thymus
thymus histone
thyroglobulin
thyroid**
thyroid cartilage
thyroid gland
thyroid hormone
thyroid-stimulating hormone
thyrotropin
thyroxin
thyroxine
tibi-
tibia
tibial
tibial nerve
tibio-
tibiofibular
tic**
-tic
tic douloureux
tick**
tidal volume
tide**
tied**
tiers**
tight junction
Tinactin
tincture

tincture of iodine
tine**
tinea**
tinea cruris
tinea pedis
tinged
tingling
tinnitus
tipped uterus
tissue
titanic**
titer
T-lymphocyte
toad skin
tocology
tocopherol
toe**
toe bones
toenail
tolbutamide
tolerance
tolerate
tolerated
tolnaftate
tome
tomography
-tomy
tone
tongue
tongue blade
tongue depressor
-tonia
tonic
tonicity
tonometer
tonsil
tonsil and adenoidectomy
tonsill-
tonsillar
tonsillectomy
tonsillitis
tonsillo-
tonus
-tony
tooth
toothache
tooth bonding
toothbrush

toothcapping
toothpaste
toothpowder
top-
tophaceous gout
tophus
topical
topo-
torn cartilage
torpor
torque
torsion
torso
torus
totally nonfunctional
total mastectomy
touch
Tourette's syndrome
tourniquet
tow**
towel
tox-
toxemia
toxi-
toxic
toxic-
toxicity
toxico-
toxicology
toxicosis
toxic shock
toxic shock syndrome
toxin
toxo-
toxoid
toxoplasmosis
trabeculae
trabecular
trace element
tracer
trache-
trachea
tracheal
trachelotomy**
tracheo-
tracheobronchial
tracheoscopy
tracheostomy

tracheotomy**
trachoma
tracing
tracked**
tract**
traction
traction splint
tractus
tragus
trail**
training
trait
TRAM
trance**
tranquilizer
trans**
trans-**
transactional analysis
transamination**
transanimation**
transdermal patch
transducer
transduction
transected
transection
transfer
transference
transferrin
transfixion
transfusion
transient situational disorder
transitional
transitory
translocation
transmission
transplant
transport molecule
transposition**
transposon**
transurethral resection of the
    prostate
transverse colon
transvestitism
trapezium
trapezius
trapezoid
trauma
trauma center

traumatic anxiety
treacle**
treadmill
treatment
tree molasses
tree sugar
trehalose
tremor
tremulous
trench mouth
trepan
trephine**
trephone**
treponema
tri-
triacylglycerol
triad
triage
trial**
triangular
Triavil
tribromoethanol
tricarboxylic acid cycle
triceps
trich
trich-
trichinosis
trichloromethane
tricho-
trichomonads
trichomonas
Trichomonas vaginalis
trichomycosis
Trichophyton
trickle**
tricuspid valve disease
tricyclic antidepressants
tricyclic compounds
trifluoperazine
triflupromazine
trigeminal nerve
trigger
triglyceride
triglycerides
trigone
trigonum
trimester
Trional

triple
triplet
trisomy
tRNA
trocar
trochanter
troche
trochlea**
trochlear**
trochlear nerve
troph-
trophic**
-trophic
tropho-
trophoblastic disease
-trophy
-tropia
tropic**
-tropic
tropical
tropical medicine
tropomyosin
troponin
trough
true rib
truncus
trunk
truss
truth serum
Trypanosoma gambiense
trypanosomiasis
trypsin
trypsins
tryptophan
tuba**
tubal**
tubal insufflation
tubal ligation
tubal pregnancy
tube
tubectomy
tuber**
tubercle
tubercul-
tuberculin
tuberculin test
tuberculo-
tuberculosis

tuberosity
tubes**
tubo-insufflation
tubo-ovarian pregnancy
tubouterine pregnancy
tubular
tubus**
Tuinal
tularemia
tumescence
tumescent
tumor
Tums
tunica
tunica albuginea
tunica dartos
tunnel
turbidity
turbinate
turgor
turista
TURP
turpentine
tussal**
tussis
tussle**
t-wave
twilight
twitch
tybamate
Tylenol
tylosin
tympanic membrane
tympanites**
tympanitis**
type
type and cross-match
typhlo-
typhoid
-typhoid
typhoid fever
typhus
typhus fever
tyroid**
tyrosine
tyrothricin
Tzanck test

U

-ular
ulcer
ulcerate
ulcerative colitis
-ulent
uln/o-
ulna**
ulnar**
ulnar nerve
ulo-
ultra-
ultrafiltrate
ultrasonic therapy
ultrasonography
ultrasound
ultraviolet therapy
-ulum
-ulus
umbilical
umbilical cord
umbilicus
unable**
uncal**
uncle**
uncompensated care
unconscious
uncontrollable
unconventional slow virus
   infections
underarm
underbite
underweight
undescended
undetermined
undifferentiated
undulent fever
unequivocal diagnosis
ungual**
unguent
ungula**
uni-
unilateral
unique**
uniquely abled
universal antidote

unknown
unofficial
unsaturated fat
unstable
unvaccinated
Upjohn
upper arm
upper extremities
upper GI series
upper respiratory infection
ur-
uracil
uran-
urano-
uranyl**
urea
-urea
uremia
uremia vesicle
uremic
uretal
ureter**
ureter-
uretero-
urethane
urethr-
urethra**
urethral
urethritis
urethro-
uretic ridge
urgency
-uria
uric-
uric acid
urico-
urin-
urinal**
urinalysis
urinary
urinary bladder
urinary tract
urinary tract infection
urination
urine

urino-
uro-
urofollitropin
urogenital
urolagnia
urological
urology
urono-
uroscopy
urticaria
use
U.S. recommended daily allowance
uter-
uteri
uterine

uterine contractant
uterine contractions
utero-
utero-ovarian varicocele
uteropelvic junction
uterus
utilization review committee
utricle
uvea**
uveal**
uveitis
uvula**
uvulae
uvular**
U wave

V

vaccin
vaccination
vaccine**
vaccinee**
vaccine therapy
vacuole
vacuum
vacuum aspiration
vag-
vagal
vagin/i-
vagina
vaginal cream
vaginal foam
vaginismus
vaginitis
vagino-
vaginolabial
vaginorectal
vago-
vague
vagus nerve
VA hospital
valence
-valence
-valent
valerian

valgus
valine
Valium**
vallum**
Valsalva's maneuver
valva**
valve**
valvotomy
valvul/o-
valvula**
valvulae**
valvular**
valvular heart disease
valvulotomy
vancomycin
vaporize
vapors
variance**
variants**
varic/o-
varicella
varicocele
varicose
varicose-valent
varicose veins
varicosity
variola

varix
varus
vas**
vas/o-
vasal**
vascul/o-
vascularity
vascular spiders
vascular system
vas deferens
vasectomy
Vaseline
vaso-
vasocongestion
vasoconstriction
vasoconstrictor
vasodilation
vasodilator
vasometer
vasopressin
vasopressor
vast**
vault
VD
vector**
vegetable albumin
vegetative state
vein
Velpeau
velum
ven/i/o-
vena**
vena cava
venae**
venereal
venereal disease
venipuncture
venography
venous**
-venous
venous disorders
venous thrombosis
ventilation
ventr/i/o-
ventral
-ventral
ventricle

ventricular
ventricular fibrillation
ventriculography
venul-
venula
venular**
venule**
venulo-
venus**
vergence**
vermi-
vermicide
vermicular
vermiform appendix
vermifuge
verruca
version
vertebr-
vertebra
vertebrae
vertebral column
vertebro-
vertex**
vertical**
verticil**
vertigo
vesica**
vesical**
vesicle**
vesico-
vesicul/o-
vesicula**
vesicular**
vessel**
vestibular nerve
vestibular system
vestibule
vestibulitis
vestigial organ
veteran's hospital
veterinarian
veterinary
veterinary medicine
viable
vial**
vibratory sensation
vibrio**

Vibrio**
vicarious
vice**
Vicks Vaporub
victimization
victor**
vidian
view
viewing instrument
vigorous exercise
vile**
villose**
villous**
villus**
Vincent's angina
vinyl
viomycin
viral**
viral diseases
viral infection
viralizing
virgin
virgins**
virile**
virilization
viroid
virology
virose**
virous**
virulent
virus**
viscera
visceral
viscid
viscous**
viscus**
vise**
visible
vision
visual

vita-
vital
vital capacity
vital signs
vitamin
vitamin deficiency
vitellin**
vitelline**
vitreous humor
vitro
vocal cords
vocal fold
voice box
void
vola**
volar**
volar arches
volatile
-volemia
volitional
volsella
volume
voluntary muscle
voluntary nervous system
-volute
vomer
vomiting
-vorous
vortex**
vox
voyeurism
vulgaris
vulsella
vulv-
vulva**
vulvar**
vulvar dystrophy
vulvitis
vulvo-

W

waist**
wait**
waiting room

walker
walleye
wandering pacemaker

ward**
warfarin
Warner Chilcott
wart**
Wassermann test
waste**
wasting
watery eyes
Watson
wax-like secretion
waxy flexibility
way**
weak**
weakness
weaning
weapon
weasand
web space
wedge resection
week**
weigh**
weight**
weight bearing
well-baby care
well-healed scar
well-woman clinic
welt
wen**
Western blot
wheal**
wheel**
wheelchair
wheezing
when**
whey**
whiplash
whiplash injury
whirlpool bath
white blood cell
white cell
whitehead
whites
white wax
whitish plaques

whitlow
WHO
whole**
whole blood
whooping cough
whorl
whorled cells
wick
wide local incision
widening
widespread
windpipe
wisdom tooth
witch hazel
withdrawal
withdrawal reflex
withdrawal symptoms
withdrawn
withering
within
Wolffian body
womb
wonder drug
wood sugar
word salad
work-up
World Health Organization
worm
worms
wound
wrap
wrench
wrenching pain
wrinkling
wrist
wrist bone
write**
writer's cramp
writhing
written orders
wrongful death
wryneck
Wyeth-Ayerst

X

xanax
xanth-
xanthene**
xanthine**
xantho-
xanthochromatic fluid
xanthoma
x-chromosomal aberration
x-chromosome
xeno-
xer-
xero-**

xerosis
xerostoma
xiph/i/o-
xiphoid process
x-linkage
x-ray
x-ray machine
x-ray technician
x-ray therapy
xylo-
xylose
xyster

Y

yaws
y-chromosome
yeast
yellow fever
yellowish discharge
yellow marrow
yoke**

yolk**
yolk sac
yolk stalk
Y-shaped scar
Y-type incision
yuppie flue

Z

Zantac
zein
Zeiss
zero**
zero-**
Z-flap
zidovudine
ZIFT/Zift
zinc
zinc ointment
zinc oxide
zo-

-zoic
-zoite
zone
zonular cataract
zonule fibers
zoo-
-zoon
zoonosis
zoster
zwieback
zyglo-
Zovirax

243

zygoma
zygomatic
zygomatic arch
zygomaticofacial nerve
zygomatic reflex
zygote

zygote intra-fallopian transfer
zyme-
-zyme
zymo-
zymogen granule